Cardiac Arrhythmias

Practical notes on interpretation and treatment

Cardiac Arrhythmias

Practical notes on interpretation and treatment

Fourth Edition

David H. Bennett MD, FRCP, FACC, FESC
Consultant Cardiologist,
Regional Cardiac Centre,
Wythenshawe Hospital, Manchester, UK

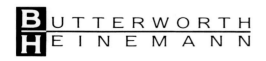

Butterworth-Heinemann Ltd
Linacre House, Jordan Hill, Oxford OX2 8DP

℟ A member of the Reed Elsevier plc group

OXFORD   LONDON   BOSTON
MUNICH   NEW DELHI   SINGAPORE   SYDNEY
TOKYO   TORONTO   WELLINGTON

First published 1981
Second edition 1985
Reprinted 1986, 1987
Third edition 1989
Reprinted 1990, 1991
Fourth edition 1993
Reprinted 1994

British Library Cataloguing in Publication Data
Bennett, David H.
  Cardiac Arrhythmias: Practical Notes on
  Interpretation and Treatment. – 4Rev. ed
  I Title
  616.1

ISBN 0 7506 1638 5

Library of Congress Cataloguing in Publication Data
Bennett, David H.
  Cardiac arrhythmias: practical notes on interpretation and
  treatment/ David H. Bennett. – 4th ed.
  p. cm.
  Includes index.
  ISBN 0 7506 1638 5
  1. Arrhythmia.   I. Title.
  [DNLM: 1. Arrhythmia – diagnosis.   2. Arrhythmia – therapy.   WG 330
  B471c 1993]
  RC685.A65B46   1993
  616.1'28–dc20
  DNLM/DLC
  For Library of Congress   93-15125
                                                              CIP

Composition by Genesis Typesetting, Laser Quay, Rochester, Kent
Printed in Great Britain at the University Press, Cambridge

Contents

Preface to the fourth edition

The purpose of this fourth edition remains the same as its predecessors: to provide a practical guide to the diagnosis, investigation and management of the main cardiac arrhythmias with particular emphasis on the problems commonly encountered in practice.

There have been many developments in the understanding and management of arrhythmias since the last edition was written some five years ago. Accordingly, the text has been extensively revised and updated.

D.H.B.

Preface to the first edition

The purpose of this book is to describe the main cardiac arrhythmias, with particular emphasis on the problems commonly encountered in their interpretation, and to discuss the practical aspects of current methods of investigation and treatment. Information of purely academic value has not been included.

This book is intended to fill the gap between those textbooks that cover only the basics of arrhythmias and those that are written for the cardiac electrophysiologist. It has been written with junior hospital doctors in mind. They receive little formal training in the management of cardiac arrhythmias and yet, because prompt action is often required, the onus of diagnosis and treatment usually falls on them. It should also be of interest to medical students, who themselves will soon be responsible for dealing with arrhythmias, to nurses working in coronary and intensive care units and to physicians who want a brief review of the practical aspects of cardiac arrhythmias.

I would like to thank the cardiac technicians, coronary care nurses and medical staff at Wythenshawe Hospital for their help. I am particularly grateful to my colleagues, Dr Colin Bray and Dr Christopher Ward.

Thanks are also due to Mrs Mary Rooney for typing the manuscript and to the Wythenshawe Hospital Medical Illustration Department.

Finally, I would like to acknowledge the distractions provided by my family, Irene, Samantha and Sally, to whom this book is dedicated.

D.H.B.

Notes

The electrocardiograms in this book have been recorded at a paper speed of 25 mm/s, unless otherwise indicated. At this speed, each large square represents 0.2 s and each small square represents 0.04 s. Heart rate (beats/minute) can therefore be calculated by dividing the number of large squares between two consecutive complexes into 300, or by dividing the number of small squares between two complexes into 1500.

Remember, when assessing a cardiac rhythm that only atrial and ventricular activity register on the surface electrocardiogram. The site of impulse formation, sequence of cardiac chamber activation and functions of the sinus node and atrioventricular junction have to be deduced from analysis of the atrial and ventricular electrograms.

A single 'rhythm strip' may be inadequate for diagnosis. Scrutiny of several ECG leads, preferably recorded simultaneously, may be necessary. For example, atrial activity is often the key to diagnosis but may not be clearly shown in all ECG leads: it is often best seen in leads II and V1.

An electrocardiogram (wherever possible a full 12-lead ECG) recorded during an arrhythmia that is of diagnostic importance should always be safely stored. This guideline which may be important to the long-term management of a patient (e.g. pacemaker implantation or anti-arrhythmic therapy) is not infrequently ignored, particularly on intensive care units!

1

Sinus rhythm

ECG characteristics   Sinus bradycardia
  P wave   Sinus tachycardia
  PR interval   Sinus arrhythmia
  QRS complex

ECG characteristics

The sinus node initiates the electrical impulse that leads to the activation of atrial and then ventricular myocardium during each heart beat. Sinus node activity itself does not register on the electrocardiogram (ECG).

P wave

Atrial activity, the P wave, is usually apparent in most ECG leads (Figure 1.1). However, sometimes the P wave is of low amplitude and it may be necessary to inspect all leads of the ECG to establish there is sinus rhythm (Figure 1.2).

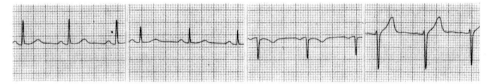

Figure 1.1 Sinus rhythm (leads I, AVF, AVR and V2). Atrial activity is clearly seen in the limb leads but is only just discernible in V2

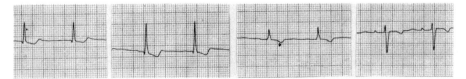

Figure 1.2 Sinus rhythm with low-amplitude P waves (leads I, II, III and V1). Atrial activity is only clearly seen in V1

Atrial activation spreads from the sinus node, which lies at the junction of the superior vena cava and right atrium, in an inferior direction towards the atrioventricular (AV) junction. The P wave, therefore, is upright in leads II, III and AVF, which face the inferior surface of the heart, and is inverted in AVR, which faces the superior heart surface (Figure 1.1). If a P wave does not have these characteristics, then, even though each ventricular complex may be preceded by a P wave, the sinus node has not activated the atria and the rhythm is abnormal (Figure 1.3).

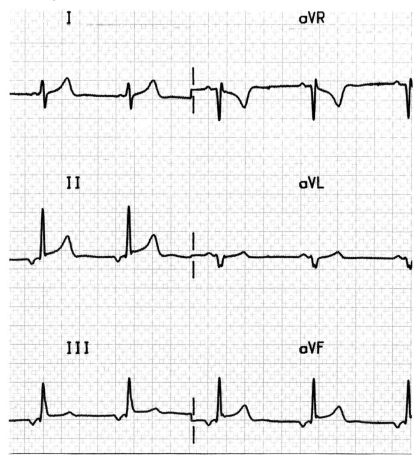

Figure 1.3 Junctional rhythm: a P wave precedes each QRS complex but is superiorly directed

PR interval

The AV node delays conduction of the atrial impulse to the ventricles. The PR interval, which is measured from the onset of the P wave to the onset of the ventricular complex, indicates the time taken for an atrial impulse to reach the ventricles. The normal PR interval ranges from 0.12 to 0.21 s. It shortens during sinus tachycardia.

QRS complex

After traversing the AV node, the activating impulse reaches the bundle of His and right and left bundle branches which rapidly conduct it to the ventricular myocardium. Ventricular activation is represented by the QRS complex which is normally less than 0.08 s in duration.

Sinus bradycardia

The definition of sinus bradycardia is sinus rhythm at a rate less than 60/minute (Figure 1.4). It may be physiological, as in athletes or during sleep, or result from acute

**Table 1.1 The characteristics of
normal sinus rhythm**

P wave:
    precedes each QRS complex
    upright in leads III, AVF
    inverted in lead AVR

PR interval:
    duration 0.12–0.21 s

QRS complex:
    duration less than 0.08 s

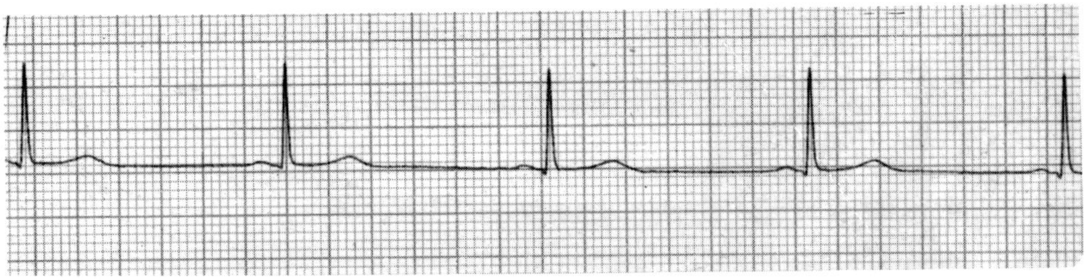

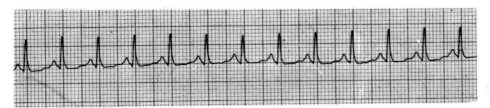

Figure 1.4 Sinus bradycardia: rate 48/minute

myocardial infarction, sick sinus syndrome or from drugs such as beta-adrenoceptor blocking drugs. Non-cardiac disorders such as myxoedema, jaundice and raised intracranial pressure can also cause sinus bradycardia.

    Atropine or pacing can increase the rate but are only necessary when sinus bradycardia causes symptoms, marked hypotension or leads to tachyarrhythmia.

Sinus tachycardia

This is defined as sinus rhythm at a rate greater than 100/minute (Figure 1.5). Exercise, anxiety or any disorder that increases sympathetic nervous system activity may cause sinus tachycardia. Occasionally it may be due to a primary disorder of the sinus node (sinus node re-entry).

    Since sinus tachycardia is usually a physiological response, there is rarely a need for specific treatment. However, if sinus tachycardia is inappropriate, the rate may be slowed by beta-adrenoceptor blocking drugs.

Figure 1.5 Sinus tachycardia during exercise (lead II): rate 150/minute

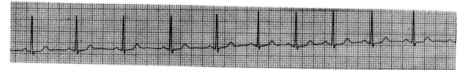

Figure 1.6 Sinus arrhythmia

At rest, the sinus node rate is seldom above 100/minute unless the patient is very ill. In contrast, atrial flutter with 2:1 AV block often leads to a heart rate of 140–160/minute and can easily be mistaken for sinus tachycardia (see Chapter 6).

Sinus arrhythmia

Normally there are only minor changes in rate during sinus rhythm. In sinus arrhythmia, which is of no pathological significance, there are alternating periods of slowing and increasing sinus node rate. Usually the rate increases during inspiration (Figure 1.6). Sinus arrhythmia is most commonly seen in the young.

Main points

- During sinus rhythm, an inferiorly directed P wave (i.e. upright in leads III and AVF) precedes each QRS complex.
- If AV conduction is normal, the duration of the PR interval will be between 0.12 and 0.21 s.
- Normal intraventricular conduction results in a QRS complex with a duration less than 0.08 s.
- In cases of apparent sinus tachycardia at rest, exclude atrial flutter or tachycardia.

Ectopic beats

Prematurity

The terms ectopic beat, extrasystole and premature contraction are, for practical purposes, synonymous. They refer to an impulse originating from the atria, AV junction (i.e. AV node plus bundle of His) or ventricles, which arises prematurely in the cardiac cycle (Figures 2.1–2.3).

Ectopic beats are by definition premature. Thus the interval between the ectopic beat and the preceding beat (i.e. the coupling interval) is shorter than the cycle length of the dominant rhythm. If this fact is forgotten, other beats with abnormal configurations such as escape beats (see Chapter 3) and intermittent bundle branch block (see Chapter 4) may be misinterpreted as ectopic beats.

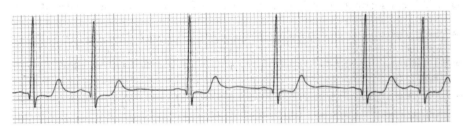

Figure 2.1 Atrial ectopic beats (second and sixth beats). The ectopic P waves differ slightly in shape from those of sinus origin

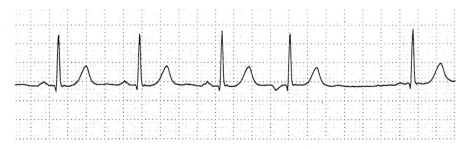

Figure 2.2 The fourth beat is a junctional ectopic beat (lead III). The junctional focus has activated the atria as well as the ventricles, resulting in an inverted P wave which precedes the QRS complex

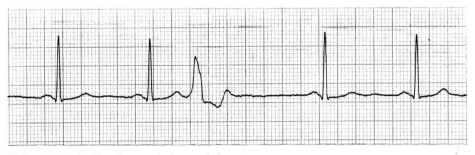

Figure 2.3 The third beat is a ventricular ectopic beat

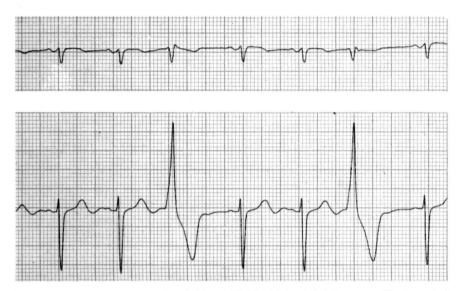

Figure 2.4 Simultaneous recording of leads V1 and V2. The third and sixth beats are unifocal ventricular ectopic beats. Their ventricular origin is not apparent in lead V1 but is obvious in V2

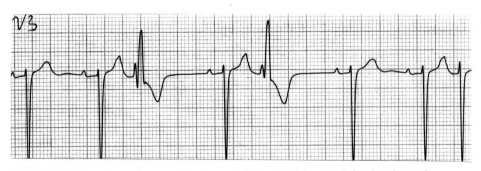

Figure 2.5 Atrial ectopic beats are superimposed on the T waves of the second, fourth and seventh ventricular complexes (lead V3). It can be seen how the T waves of these beats are modified by comparing them with the T wave of the first and sixth ventricular complexes which are not followed by an atrial ectopic. The first two atrial ectopic beats are conducted with right bundle branch block

The site of origin of an ectopic beat can be determined by careful examination of the ECG. A single rhythm strip may be inadequate. Scrutiny of simultaneous recordings of several ECG leads is often necessary to detect the diagnostic clues (Figures 2.4 and 2.5).

Atrial ectopic beats

P wave

An atrial ectopic beat results in a premature P wave. The source and hence direction of atrial activation will differ from that during sinus rhythm so a premature P wave will often differ in shape to a P wave of sinus node origin (Figure 2.1).

Because atrial ectopic beats are premature, they may be superimposed on and thus deform the T wave of the preceding beat. Careful examination of the ECG is essential to detect ectopic P waves; often, lead V1 is the best lead (Figures 2.5 and 2.6).

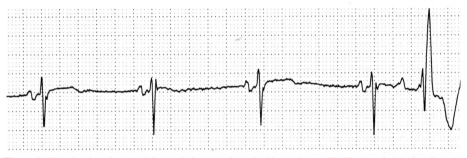

Figure 2.6 The last beat is an atrial ectopic beat conducted with 1st degree AV block and right bundle branch block

AV and intraventricular conduction

Usually the AV junction and bundle branches will conduct an atrial ectopic beat to the ventricles in the same manner as if the sinus node had activated the atria. Thus the PR interval and QRS complex of the ectopic beat will be identical with those during sinus rhythm (Figure 2.1). If the QRS complex during sinus rhythm shows bundle branch block, then so will the QRS complex in the ectopic beat.

Sometimes however, atrial ectopic beats, especially those that arise very early in the cardiac cycle, may encounter either an AV junction or a bundle branch which has not yet recovered from conduction of the last atrial impulse and is, therefore, partially or completely refractory to excitation. Partial and complete refractoriness of the AV junction will result in prolongation of the PR interval and blocked atrial ectopic beats, respectively (Figures 2.6–2.8). Blocked atrial ectopics have been erroneously taken as an indication for cardiac pacing!

Partial or complete refractoriness of one or other bundle branch (it is usually the right bundle) will correspondingly lead to partial or complete bundle branch block (Figure 2.7). This phenomenon of functional bundle branch block is referred to by some as 'phasic aberrant intraventricular conduction'. The resultant QRS complexes are broad and can therefore be confused with ventricular ectopic beats if the premature P wave preceding the ventricular complex is not detected.

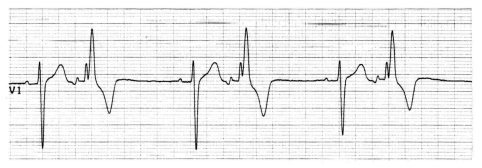

Figure 2.7 Atrial ectopic beats follow each sinus beat and are conducted with right bundle branch block

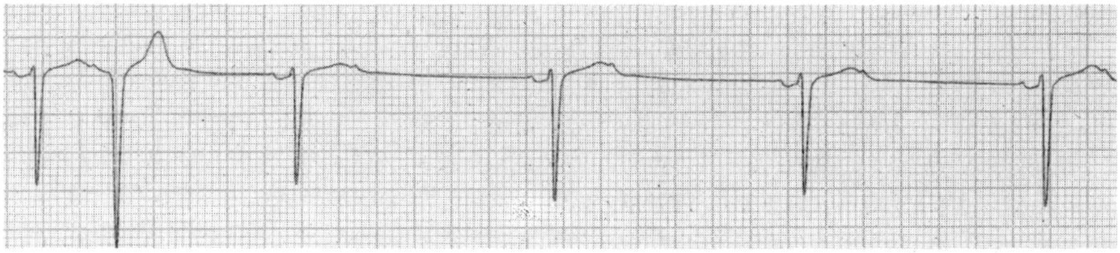

Figure 2.8 Lead V1. Atrial ectopic beats are superimposed on the T wave of each ventricular complex. The first atrial ectopic is conducted with partial left branch block. The other atrial ectopic beats are not conducted to the ventricles

Table 2.1 Characteristics of atrial ectopic beats

The P wave:
> will be premature
> may be superimposed on and distort the preceding T wave
> will usually be followed by a normal QRS complex
> may sometimes not be conducted to the ventricles or be
>   conducted with a bundle branch block pattern

Significance

Atrial ectopic beats are often benign and do occur in subjects with normal hearts. However, if they are frequent they may clinically mimic atrial fibrillation and may herald its onset.

AV junctional ectopic beats

AV junctional beats used to be called 'nodal' beats. It is now recognized that at least part of the AV node is not capable of pacemaker activity and that it is not possible to distinguish between beats of AV nodal and His bundle origin. Hence the more general term 'AV junction'. AV junctional ectopic beats are not as common as atrial or ventricular ectopics. Treatment is rarely necessary.

ECG appearance

AV junctional ectopic beats are recognized by a premature QRS complex which is similar in appearance to that occurring in sinus rhythm. The junctional focus may activate the atria as well as the ventricles, leading to a retrograde P wave (i.e. negative in leads II, III and AVF). The retrograde P wave may precede, follow or be buried within the QRS complex, depending on the relative speeds of conduction of the premature junctional impulse to the ventricles and to the atria (Figure 2.2).

Ventricular ectopic beats

These result in a premature ventricular complex which is broad (>0.12 s), bizarre in shape and, in contrast to atrial ectopic beats, will obviously not be preceded by an ectopic P wave (Figures 2.3 and 2.4).

Table 2.2 Characteristics of ventricular ectopic beats

With ventricular ectopic beats the QRS complex:
    will be premature
    will be broad (>0.12 s)
    will be abnormal in shape
    will not be preceded by a premature P wave

ECG appearance

A ventricular ectopic beat does not activate the ventricles via the specialized, rapidly conducting tissues. The abnormal shape and prolonged duration of the ventricular complex reflect the abnormal course and consequent slowing of ventricular activation.

Several terms are used to describe different types of ventricular ectopic beats:

Focus

Ectopic beats with the same shape and coupling intervals are assumed to arise from the same focus and are termed unifocal, whereas differing shapes and coupling intervals imply more than one focus, i.e. multifocal (Figures 2.4 and 2.9).

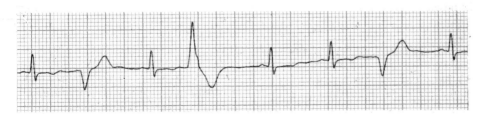

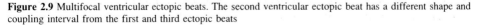

Figure 2.9 Multifocal ventricular ectopic beats. The second ventricular ectopic beat has a different shape and coupling interval from the first and third ectopic beats

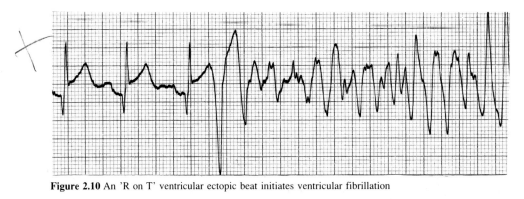

Figure 2.10 An 'R on T' ventricular ectopic beat initiates ventricular fibrillation

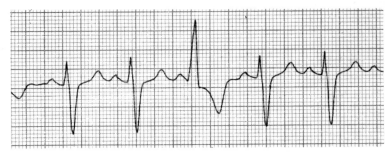

Figure 2.11 The third beat is an end-diastolic ventricular ectopic beat. It is preceded by a normally timed P wave

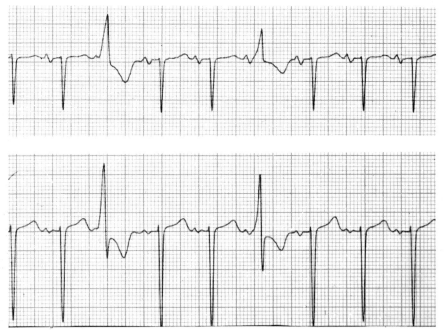

Figure 2.12 Simultaneous recording of leads V1 and V2. Two end-diastolic ventricular ectopic beats, the second mimicking the Wolff–Parkinson–White syndrome

Timing

Beats that occur very early in the cardiac cycle will be superimposed on the T wave of the preceding beat and are described as 'R on T' (Figure 2.10). Most episodes of ventricular fibrillation and many episodes of ventricular tachycardia are initiated by 'R on T' ectopics; though by no means do all 'R on T' ectopic beats precipitate these arrhythmias.

A ventricular ectopic beat that occurs only slightly prematurely in the cardiac cycle may fall, by chance, immediately after a P wave initiated by sinus node activity. The P wave will therefore, in contrast to an atrial ectopic beat, be normal in timing and configuration. This is referred to as an 'end-diastolic' ventricular ectopic beat (Figures 2.11, 2.12).

Usually there is a pause after a ventricular ectopic beat. When there is no such pause and the ectopic beat is thus sandwiched between two normal beats, the ectopic beat is said to be 'interpolated' (Figure 2.13).

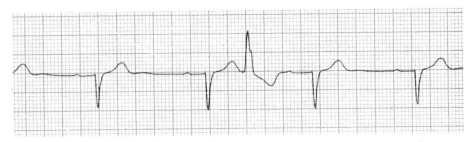

Figure 2.13 Interpolated ventricular beat. The subsequent PR interval is prolonged owing to retrograde concealed conduction

Quantification

Ventricular ectopic beats are often quantified by the number occurring each minute.

When an ectopic beat follows each sinus beat, the term bigeminy is applied (Figure 2.14). If an ectopic follows a pair of normal beats there is trigeminy. When two ectopics occur in succession (Figure 2.15) they are referred to as a couplet. A salvo refers to more than two ectopic beats in succession (see Chapter 5).

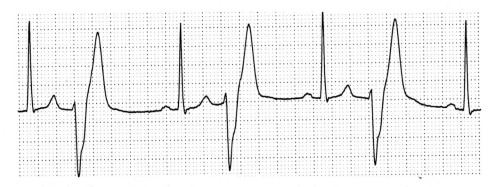

Figure 2.14 Ventricular bigeminy

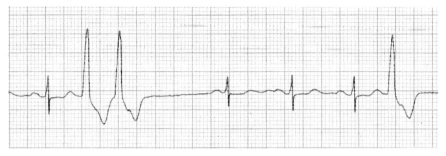

Figure 2.15 The first sinus beat is followed by a couplet of ventricular ectopic beats

Atrial activity

The pattern of atrial activity following a ventricular ectopic beat depends on whether the AV junction transmits the ventricular impulse to the atria. If this occurs the result is an inverted P wave which is often superimposed on, and may therefore be concealed by, the ventricular ectopic beat (Figure 2.16). When the AV junction does not transmit the ventricular impulse to the atria, atrial activity proceeds independently of ventricular activity; it is only in these cases that a ventricular impulse is followed by a full compensatory pause, i.e. the lengths of the cycles before and after the ectopic beat will equal twice the sinus cycle length (see Figures 2.3 and 2.4).

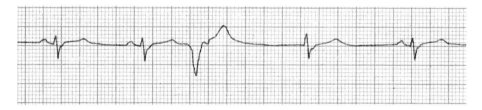

Figure 2.16 The third beat is a ventricular ectopic beat which has been conducted back to the atria, resulting in an inverted P wave (lead AVF). (The ectopic beat is followed by a junctional escape beat)

Sometimes a ventricular impulse only partially penetrates the AV junction. The subsequent impulse arising from sinus node activation may find the AV junction partially refractory and be conducted with a prolonged PR interval (Figure 2.13). This phenomenon of 'retrograde concealed conduction' often occurs following interpolated ventricular extrasystoles.

Parasystole

As stated above, unifocal ventricular ectopic beats have a constant coupling interval. Ventricular parasystole, which is uncommon, is an exception to this rule. In this arrhythmia a ventricular ectopic focus discharges regularly and is undisturbed by the dominant rhythm. It will capture the ventricles provided the ectopic discharge does not occur when the ventricles have just been activated by the dominant rhythm and are therefore refractory. Thus ventricular parasystole (Figure 2.17) is characterized by a variable coupling interval, inter-ectopic intervals which are multiples of a common factor

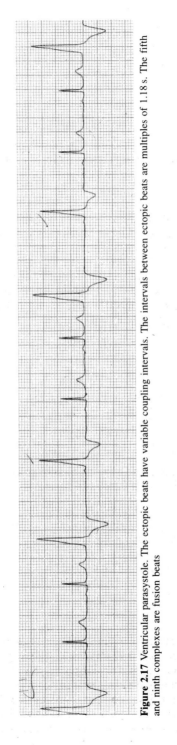

Figure 2.17 Ventricular parasystole. The ectopic beats have variable coupling intervals. The intervals between ectopic beats are multiples of 1.18 s. The fifth and ninth complexes are fusion beats

and, because the ventricles may by chance be simultaneously activated by both ectopic and normal pacemakers, fusion beats (i.e. complexes that are in appearance a fusion between normal and ectopic beats).

Causes and significance of ventricular ectopic beats

Causes include acute myocardial infarction, myocardial ischaemia or damage caused by previous infarction, myocarditis, cardiomyopathy, mitral valve prolapse, valvular heart disease and digoxin toxicity.

Occasional ventricular ectopic beats at rest and even frequent unifocal ectopic beats on exercise occur in otherwise normal individuals and are not necessarily pathological or of prognostic significance. The frequency of ectopic beats in the adult population increases with age.

In contrast, 'complex' ventricular ectopic beats – i.e. frequent, multifocal, 'R on T' or those that occur in salvos – are infrequently found in the absence of cardiac disease and are associated with an increased cardiovascular mortality.

In chronic ischaemic heart disease, there is a correlation between severity of left ventricular damage and frequency of ventricular ectopic beats. Recent evidence, however, points to the presence of ectopic beats as an additional and independent risk factor but there is no evidence to show that suppression of ectopic beats by anti-arrhythmic therapy improves prognosis. Indeed, in a recent study of patients with ventricular ectopic beats after myocardial infarction, several anti-arrhythmic drugs increased mortality.

Usually, ectopic beats do not cause symptoms. Some patients, however, experience distressing symptoms. They may be upset by the irregularity caused by premature beats or by the compensatory pause or 'thump' caused by increased myocardial contractility associated with the post-ectopic beat. In this minority of patients anti-arrhythmic therapy may be necessary for symptomatic purposes.

The significance of ventricular ectopic beats in acute myocardial infarction is discussed in Chapter 11.

Main points

- Ectopic beats are premature and therefore have a coupling interval shorter than the cycle length of the dominant rhythm.
- The P waves of atrial ectopic beats are often superimposed on and distort the preceding T wave and can easily be missed. They are usually best seen in lead Vl.
- Atrial ectopic beats may sometimes not be conducted to the ventricles or may be conducted with a bundle branch block pattern.
- Ventricular ectopic beats cause premature, broad and bizarrely shaped QRS complexes. They are only followed by a full compensatory pause if they are not conducted to the atria.
- Chronic ventricular ectopic beats which are frequent, multifocal, 'R on T' or occur in salvos are associated with an increased cardiovascular mortality but there is no evidence to show that their suppression improves prognosis.

Escape beats

Timing

When the dominant pacemaker fails to discharge, escape beats may arise from subsidiary pacemaker tissue. In contrast to ectopic beats, escape beats are always late, i.e. the coupling interval is greater than the cycle length of the dominant rhythm (Figures 3.1 and 3.3). Distinction between escape and ectopic beats is important because the former suggest impaired pacemaker function. Escape beats themselves require no treatment. If treatment is necessary, it is to accelerate the basic rhythm.

Origins

Escape beats usually arise from the AV junction (Figures 3.1–3.3); less commonly, they originate from the ventricles. The ventricular complexes of junctional escape beats are similar to those during normal rhythm. Ventricular escape beats have a similar configuration to ventricular ectopic beats (Figures 3.4 and 3.5).

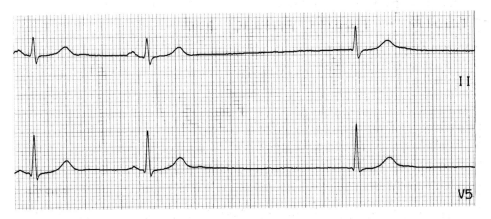

Figure 3.1 The third ventricular complex is a junctional escape beat

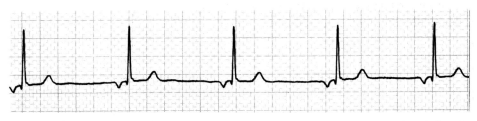

Figure 3.2 Junctional escape rhythm (lead II). The junctional focus has also activated the atria as indicated by the inverted P wave preceding each QRS complex

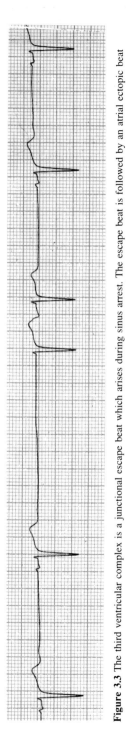

Figure 3.3 The third ventricular complex is a junctional escape beat which arises during sinus arrest. The escape beat is followed by an atrial ectopic beat

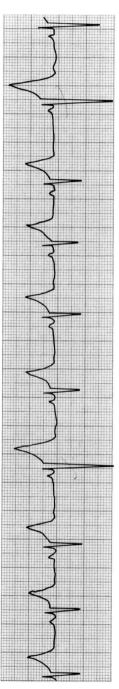

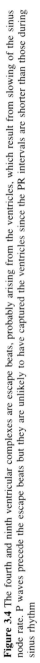

Figure 3.4 The fourth and ninth ventricular complexes are escape beats, probably arising from the ventricles, which result from slowing of the sinus node rate. P waves precede the escape beats but they are unlikely to have captured the ventricles since the PR intervals are shorter than those during sinus rhythm

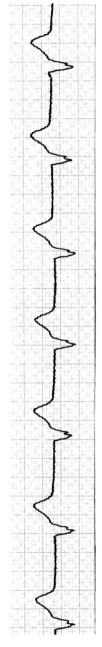

Figure 3.5 Ventricular escape rhythm

Main points

- In contrast to ectopic beats, the coupling interval of escape beats is greater than the cycle length of the dominant rhythm.
- As with ectopic beats, the configuration of escape beats indicates whether they are of supraventricular or ventricular origin.
- Escape beats should not be suppressed by drugs.

Bundle branch blocks

The bundle of His divides into left and right bundle branches. The left bundle branch has two main subdivisions: the anterior and posterior fascicles. These specialized intra-ventricular conducting tissues facilitate the rapid activation of the left and right ventricles.

Right bundle branch block

ECG appearance

In right bundle branch block, there is delay in activation of the right ventricle while septal and left ventricular activation proceed normally (Figure 4.1). Delayed right ventricular activation results in:

1. An increase in duration of the QRS complex (>0.12 s).
2. A secondary R wave in leads facing the right ventricle (Vl and V2).
3. A broad S wave in left ventricular leads, especially lead I.

Partial right bundle branch block results in a similar ECG appearance but the QRS duration is 0.11 s or less.

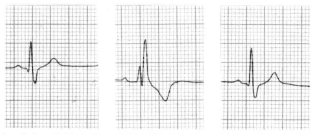

Figure 4.1 Right bundle branch block (leads I, V1, V6). There is an M-shaped complex in Vl and a deep slurred S wave in leads I and V6

Causes and significance

Right bundle branch block may be an isolated congenital lesion. It often occurs in congenital heart disease, in other causes of right ventricular hypertrophy or strain and where there is myocardial damage. Right bundle branch block is common when there is disease of the specialized conducting tissues.

Supraventricular extrasystoles and tachycardias may encounter a right bundle branch which is refractory to excitation (i.e. phasic aberrant intraventricular conduction) and be conducted to the ventricles with a right bundle branch block pattern.

Based on limited data, neither pre-existing nor acquired right bundle branch block are of poor prognostic significance.

Left bundle branch block

ECG appearance

In left bundle branch block, activation of the interventricular septum is in the opposite direction to normal, being initiated by impulses arising from the right bundle branch. Thus:

1. The initial small negative Q wave normally seen in left ventricular leads (V5, V6, I and AVL) is replaced by a larger positive R wave.
2. Activation of the left ventricle will be delayed, resulting in a secondary R wave in left ventricular leads and prolongation of the duration of the QRS complex (>0.12 s).
3. The primary and secondary R waves produce an M-shaped ventricular complex in left ventricular leads (Figure 4.2). (In contrast, right bundle branch block produces an M-shaped ventricular complex in right ventricular leads.)

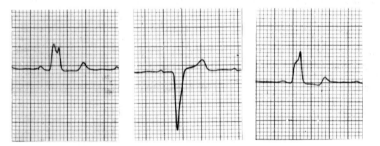

Figure 4.2 Left bundle branch block (leads I, V1, V6). There is an M-shaped complex in I and V6. The QS complex in V1 is also characteristic of left bundle branch block

Partial left bundle branch block has a similar ECG appearance to complete left bundle branch block, but the QRS duration is 0.10 or 0.11 s.

Causes and significance

Causes include myocardial damage due to coronary artery disease or cardiomyopathy, and severe left ventricular hypertrophy.

Like right bundle branch block, left bundle branch block can be caused by disease of the specialized conduction tissues. The pattern can also occur as a result of phasic aberrant intraventricular conduction. Rarely, left bundle branch block may occur in an otherwise normal heart.

Left bundle branch block can be intermittent (Figure 4.3).

Recently acquired left bundle branch block indicates the patient is at a significantly increased risk of sudden death.

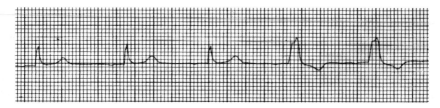

Figure 4.3 Intermittent left bundle branch block (lead AVL)

Left anterior and posterior fascicular blocks

The anterior and posterior fascicles of the left bundle branch conduct impulses to the anterosuperior and posteroinferior regions of the left ventricle, respectively.

Block can occur in either anterior or posterior fascicles and is known as fascicular block or hemiblock. Left anterior and posterior fascicular blocks are common in conduction tissue disease (see Chapter 9).

Diagnosis of the fascicular blocks is based on the hexaxial reference system.

Hexaxial reference system

The hexaxial reference system is a method of displaying the orientation of the six ECG limb leads to the heart in the frontal plane (Figure 4.4). For example, a superiorly directed impulse will move away from leads II, III and AVF, producing a negative wave in these leads, and towards AVL, producing a positive wave in this lead.

The direction of an impulse can be expressed by the number of degrees clockwise (positive) or anti-clockwise (negative) of lead I, which is the zero reference point. For example, an impulse towards lead AVL has an axis of −30° and an impulse towards lead III has an axis of +120° (Figure 4.4).

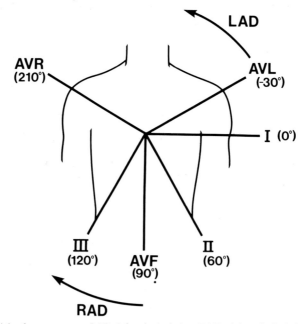

Figure 4.4 Hexaxial reference system. LAD, left axis deviation; RAD, right axis deviation

Mean frontal QRS axis

The mean frontal QRS axial describes the dominant or average direction of the various electrical forces that develop during ventricular activation. Normally, the mean frontal QRS axis lies between AVL (i.e. −30°) and AVF (i.e. +90°).

If the axis is anti-clockwise, or to the left of AVL (i.e. < −30°), it is termed abnormal left axis deviation. If the axis is clockwise, or to the right of AVF (i.e. > +90°), there is right axis deviation.

Using the hexaxial reference system, the mean frontal QRS axis may be calculated to within a few degrees. However, this degree of precision is unnecessary. It is easier to diagnose left and right axis deviation from a simple rule of thumb, as follows.

In left axis deviation, lead I is predominantly positive and both leads II and III are predominantly negative (Figure 4.5). Contrary to some older texts, both II and III must be predominantly negative, i.e. if in lead II the S wave is smaller than the R wave, abnormal left axis deviation is not present (Figure 4.6). If lead II is equiphasic, there is borderline left axis deviation (Figure 4.6).

In right axis deviation, lead I is predominantly negative and both leads II and III are predominantly positive (Figure 4.7).

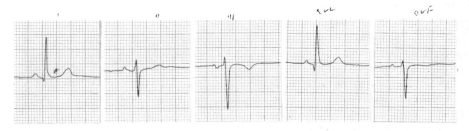

Figure 4.5 Left axis deviation due to left anterior fascicular block (leads I, II, III, AVL, AVF)

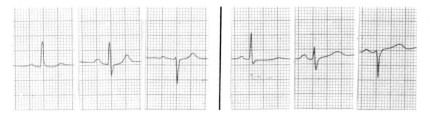

Figure 4.6 Leads I, II, III from two patients. In the first, the mean frontal QRS axis is normal. In the second, lead II is equiphasic and thus there is borderline left axis deviation

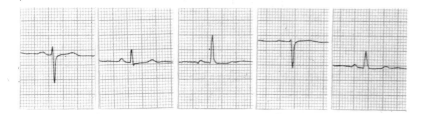

Figure 4.7 Right axis deviation due to left posterior fascicular block (leads I, II, III, AVL, AVF)

Left anterior fascicular block

Block in the anterior fascicle of the left bundle branch causes delay in activation of the anterosuperior portion of the left ventricle. Initial left ventricular activation will be via the posterior fascicle to the posteroinferior region and will therefore be directed inferiorly and to the right. This results in an initial positive deflection R wave in inferiorly orientated leads (II, III and AVF) and in an initial negative deflection Q wave in the lateral leads (I and AVL) (Figure 4.5).

The anterosuperior region will be activated by conduction from the posteroinferior region. The resultant wave will, therefore, be superiorly directed (R wave in I and AVL; S in II, III and AVF). Because conduction is through ordinary myocardium rather than the specialized conducting tissues, it will be relatively slow. As a result, activation of the anterosuperior region will be delayed and consequently unopposed by activity from the rest of the ventricles. Thus the resultant superiorly directed wave is larger than the initial inferiorly directed wave and the mean frontal QRS axis will also be superiorly directed, i.e. there will be left axis deviation.

Left anterior fascicular block is a common cause of left axis deviation. The other cause is inferior myocardial infarction (Figure 4.8).

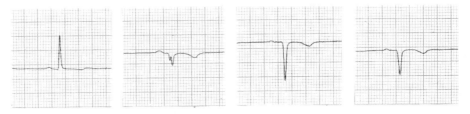

Figure 4.8 Inferior myocardial infarction (leads I, II, III, AVF). There is left axis deviation but not left anterior fascicular block

To diagnose left anterior fascicular block, two criteria must be satisfied:

1. There must be left axis deviation, i.e. lead I must be predominantly positive and leads II and III predominantly negative.
2. The initial direction of ventricular activation must be inferior and to the right, i.e. there must be an initial R wave in leads II, III and AVF.

Left posterior fascicular block

In left posterior fascicular block, activation of the posteroinferior portion of the left ventricle is delayed. As a result, there will be an initial positive R wave in leads I and AVL and an initial negative Q wave in leads II, III and AVF; and there will be right axis deviation, i.e. lead I will be predominantly negative and leads II and III predominantly positive (Figure 4.7).

A diagnosis of left posterior fascicular block can only be made in the absence of other causes of right axis deviation such as right ventricular hypertrophy or strain, or a young patient with an asthenic build.

Main points

- Complete bundle branch block prolongs QRS duration to 0.12 s or greater. In incomplete block, QRS duration is 0.10–0.11 s.
- In abnormal left axis deviation, lead I is predominantly positive and both leads II and III are predominantly negative.
- In right axis deviation, lead I is predominantly negative and leads II and III positive.
- The criteria for left anterior hemiblock are left axis deviation together with a small, initial R wave in leads II and AVF.
- Left posterior hemiblock should be considered when there is right axis deviation in the absence of its other causes, e.g. right ventricular hypertrophy or strain.

Ventricular tachycardias

Ventricular tachycardia is defined as four or more ventricular ectopic beats in rapid succession (Figure 5.1). Ventricular tachycardias vary in rate, duration and frequency of recurrence. The arrhythmia may sometimes progress to ventricular fibrillation or, if sustained, may cause shock, whereas in some circumstances it may be well tolerated with few or no symptoms.

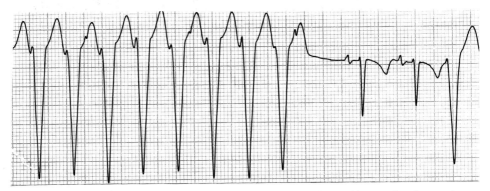

Figure 5.1 Ventricular tachycardia: a series of ventricular ectopic beats followed by two sinus beats and a single ventricular ectopic beat

Heart muscle damage resulting from coronary heart disease or from cardiomyopathy is the usual cause of the arrhythmia.

There are two main types of ventricular tachycardia: monomorphic and polymorphic.

Monomorphic ventricular tachycardia

This is the commonest form of ventricular tachycardia. The tachycardia is defined as sustained if either its duration is greater than 30 s or if it has to be terminated by cardioversion or by pacing in less than 30 s because of severe hypotension. Non-sustained tachycardia ceases spontaneously in less than 30 s.

ECG characteristics

The arrhythmia consists of a rapid succession of ventricular ectopic beats each with the same appearance, hence the term monomorphic (Figures 5.1–5.3). As with single ventricular ectopic beats, the complexes will be abnormal in shape, and the duration of each complex will be more than 0.12 s and usually greater than 0.14 s. The rhythm is regular unless there are capture beats (see below) which cause minor irregularities in the rhythm. The rate ranges from 120 to 250 beats/minute.

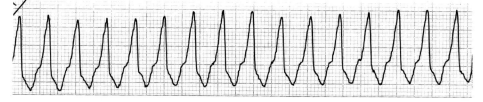

Figure 5.2 Ventricular tachycardia. There is a rapid regular succession of broad complexes

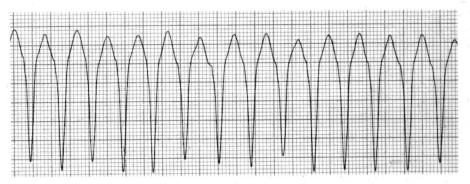

Figure 5.3 Ventricular tachycardia (lead V1)

Atrial activity during ventricular tachycardia

With many ventricular tachycardias, the sinus node continues to initiate atrial activity which is therefore independent of and slower than ventricular activity (Figure 5.4).

In others, the AV node conducts the ventricular impulses to the atria so an inverted P wave follows each ventricular complex. The superimposed terminal portion of the ventricular complex often conceals the retrogradely conducted P wave (Figure 5.5). Rarely second-degree block may occur at the AV junction so only some ventricular impulses are conducted to the atria.

Identification of independent atrial activity during tachycardia excludes an origin at AV node level or above and is thus an important pointer in distinguishing ventricular tachycardia from supraventricular tachycardia with broad ventricular complexes. There may be direct or indirect evidence of independent atrial activity.

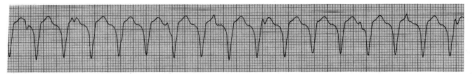

Figure 5.4 Ventricular tachycardia with direct evidence of independent atrial activity. P waves, separated by intervals of 0.75 s, can be seen after the 1st, 3rd, 6th, 8th, 10th, 13th, 15th and 17th ventricular complexes

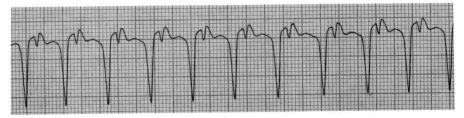

Figure 5.5 Ventricular tachycardia (lead AVF) with retrograde atrial activation. Each ventricular complex can be seen to be followed by an inverted P wave

Direct evidence of independent atrial activity

P waves at a slower rate than and dissociated from ventricular activity are direct evidence of independent atrial activity (Figure 5.4). Inevitably, some P waves will be concealed by superimposed ventricular complexes. Furthermore, not all leads will clearly show atrial activity. A rhythm strip is often inadequate and scrutiny of a simultaneous recording of several different leads may be necessary. Sometimes there will be doubt whether small waves on the ECG during tachycardia are caused by atrial activity. If they are, they will be separated by similar intervals, or multiples of that interval.

Indirect evidence of independent atrial activity

Capture or fusion beats are indirect evidence of atrial activity. Just one is sufficient to confirm ventricular tachycardia.

   Capture beats occur when the timing of an atrial impulse during ventricular tachycardia is such that it can be transmitted via the AV junction and activate the ventricles before the next discharge from the ventricular focus. The resultant ventricular complex will be normal in shape and duration and will occur slightly earlier than the next ventricular ectopic beat would have been expected (Figure 5.6).

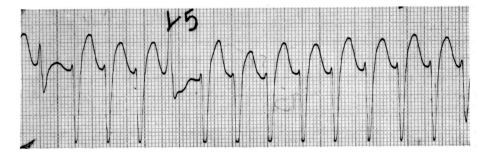

Figure 5.6 Ventricular tachycardia (lead V5). The fifth complex is a capture beat and the first complex is a fusion beat

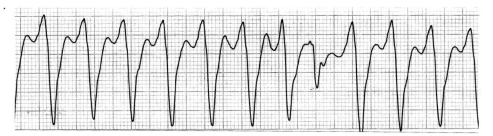

Figure 5.7 Ventricular tachycardia. The eighth complex is a fusion beat

Fusion beats are caused by a similar process. However, the atrial impulse activates the ventricles slightly later in the cardiac cycle leading to simultaneous activation of the ventricles by the transmitted atrial impulse and the ventricular focus. The result is a ventricular complex which in appearance is a fusion between a normal QRS complex and a ventricular ectopic beat (Figures 5.6 and 5.7).

Table 5.1 Characteristics of monomorphic ventricular tachycardia

Regular rhythm
Broad complexes (at least 0.12 s and usually more than 0.14 s)
Ventricular complexes of uniform appearance
Independent P waves may be present
Capture or fusion beats may be present

Causes of monomorphic ventricular tachycardia

Ventricular tachycardia is most often the result of myocardial damage from coronary heart disease or from cardiomyopathy. Table 5.2 lists the main causes.

Table 5.2 Causes of ventricular tachycardia

Acute myocardial infarction or ischaemia
Past myocardial infarction
Dilated cardiomyopathy
Hypertrophic cardiomyopathy
Myocarditis
Arrhythmogenic right ventricular dysplasia
Mitral valve prolapse
Valvular heart disease
Repair of tetralogy of Fallot
Idiopathic

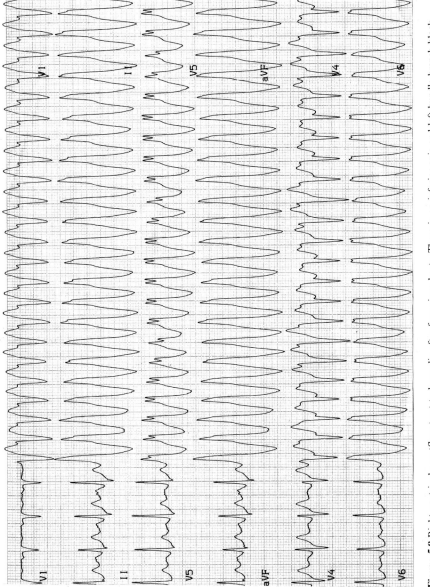

Figure 5.8 Right ventricular outflow tract tachycardia after four sinus beats. There is an inferior axis and left bundle branch block configuration

Distinctive forms of ventricular tachycardia

Right ventricular outflow tract tachycardia

This tachycardia has a characteristic ECG appearance which reflects its origin in the right ventricular outflow tract. Because the origin is in the right ventricle, the ventricular complexes are similar to those seen during left bundle branch block; and because the impulse spreads inferiorly from the outflow tract there is an inferior frontal QRS axis, i.e. right axis deviation (Figure 5.8).

Typically, the tachycardia is provoked by effort and is non-sustained. There is usually no evidence of structural cardiac disease.

Arrhythmogenic right ventricular dysplasia

Ventricular tachycardia arises from the right ventricle whose impaired function can be demonstrated by echocardiography or by angiocardiography. Sometimes only localized areas of the ventricle are affected rather than generalized dysfunction. There is little or no left ventricular impairment.

Complexes during tachycardia usually have a left bundle branch block configuration. During sinus rhythm, there is often T wave inversion or other repolarization abnormality in leads V1 to V3. Patients are usually young and the arrhythmia is often induced by exercise.

Fascicular tachycardia

This is an uncommon ventricular tachycardia which arises from the region of the posterior fascicle of the left bundle branch. Usually there is no structural heart disease.

The ventricular complexes are of relatively short duration (0.12 s), sometimes leading to confusion with supraventricular tachycardia. Their configuration is similar to right bundle branch, except there is usually a small Q wave rather than a primary R wave; and there is left axis deviation (Figure 5.9).

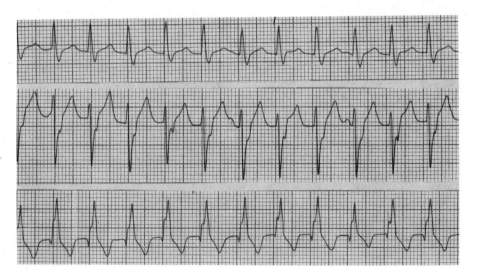

Figure 5.9 Fascicular tachycardia (leads I, II and V1). Independent atrial activity can be seen in lead II

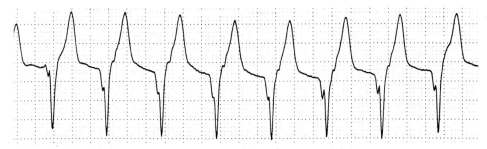

Figure 5.10 Accelerated idioventricular rhythm

Accelerated idioventricular rhythm

Monomorphic ventricular tachycardia with a rate less than 120 beats/minute is termed accelerated idioventricular rhythm or slow ventricular tachycardia (Figure 5.10). It is usually encountered during acute myocardial infarction. Treatment is unnecessary.

Mechanisms of ventricular tachycardias

There are two main types of mechanism that cause tachycardias. One is re-entry: this is the commonest mechanism for ventricular tachycardia. The other is enhanced automaticity which may be spontaneous or triggered.

Re-entry

Two conditions are necessary for a re-entrant tachycardia to occur. The first is the presence of a potential circuit made up of two pathways of tissue with differing electrical characteristics. The second is transient or permanent block in one direction in one of the pathways so an impulse can be conducted along one pathway and return in the opposite direction via the other pathway, thereby re-entering the circuit. The activating impulse is repeatedly conducted around the circuit, exciting the surrounding myocardium at a rapid rate.

In ventricular tachycardia, fibrosis or ischaemia may cause delay in activation and hence recovery of an area of myocardium. Tachycardia results when a premature beat arrives at the abnormal area to find it is refractory to excitation following the last heartbeat. The impulse is conducted around the damaged area by the adjacent normally responsive myocardium. By the time the impulse has circumvented the damaged area, the abnormal myocardium has become excitable again and conducts the impulse in the opposite direction giving rise to a re-entrant circuit. Perpetuation of this process results in ventricular tachycardia.

Enhanced automaticity

Damage or disease can result in a group of myocardial cells acquiring enhanced automaticity, i.e. the cells discharge at a higher rate than the sinus node, taking over control of the heart rhythm. Enhanced automaticity can either be spontaneous or be triggered by after-depolarizations which lead to early reactivation of the myocardium.

Initiation of tachycardia

A re-entrant circuit or focus of enhanced automaticity provide the substrate for ventricular tachycardia. Initiation of the arrhythmia is usually triggered by an ectopic beat. Ischaemia, sympathetic nervous system activity or electrolyte imbalance may influence the arrhythmia substrate and may account for a tachycardia occurring at a particular time.

Investigations

The nature and extent of investigations has to be tailored to the individual clinical situation. The aims should be to identify the cause, which may well have therapeutic or prognostic significance, and to assess the role and efficacy of any therapy that may be indicated.

12-Lead electrocardiogram

Whenever possible, a 12-lead electrocardiogram during tachycardia should be recorded and saved. It may point to the origin of the tachycardia. Furthermore, if electrophysiological studies are to be carried out, it is important to know that a tachycardia induced during the study has the same morphology and is therefore the same arrhythmia as has occurred spontaneously. Obviously, if the tachycardia leads to severe hypotension and the immediate need for cardioversion, it may not be possible to obtain a full ECG.

An ECG during sinus rhythm may reveal the cause of tachycardia, e.g. demonstrating myocardial infarction.

Imaging

Echocardiography may help establish the cause of the arrhythmia. For example, by demonstrating dilated or hypertrophic cardiomyopathy; or by showing dilatation of the right ventricle but normal left ventricular function, thereby pointing to right ventricular dysplasia.

Sometimes, cardiac catheterization may be necessary, particularly if acute ischaemia might be the cause of the arrhythmia or if surgery is contemplated.

Ambulatory electrocardiography

Ambulatory electrocardiography will help assess the frequency and duration of episodes of ventricular tachycardia and the effect of therapy in those patients who have had frequent episodes.

Occasionally, ventricular tachycardia arises during bradycardia and this may be revealed by ambulatory electrocardiography. Prevention of bradycardia will often prevent ventricular tachycardia.

Exercise testing

Exercise-induced tachycardia is common. An exercise test can be useful in its diagnosis and assessment of therapy.

Most anti-arrhythmic drugs can in some patients be pro-arrhythmic (see Chapter 12). A pro-arrhythmic effect may only be apparent during exercise. As a rule, patients who receive long-term therapy to prevent ventricular tachycardia should undergo exercise testing.

Electrophysiological study

Stimulation of the ventricles with precisely timed single or double premature stimuli will often induce ventricular tachycardia in patients who are prone to this arrhythmia. Drug therapy which then prevents reinduction of the arrhythmia or at least increases the cycle length during tachycardia by over 100 ms has been shown to have a favourable effect on prognosis. Serial testing may be necessary to identify an effective drug. Sometimes all anti-arrhythmic drugs will be found to be ineffective.

There are, however, some reservations about the predictive value of electrophysiological testing. The more aggressive the stimulation protocol in terms of the number of stimuli and the rate of stimulation, the easier it is to induce a ventricular arrhythmia. It is not clear which stimulation protocol has the best predictive accuracy. There is doubt about the significance of induction of non-sustained ventricular tachycardia. Furthermore, it does not necessarily follow that the oral preparation of a drug that has proved effective when given intravenously during an electrophysiological test will prevent spontaneous ventricular arrhythmias. Amiodarone may prevent spontaneous ventricular tachycardia and yet the arrhythmia may still be inducible, though usually at a relatively slow rate, at electrophysiological testing.

Signal-averaged electrocardiography

Late potentials are low voltage, high frequency signals in the terminal portion of the QRS complex. They indicate an area of delayed myocardial activation and are commonly found in patients subject to ventricular tachycardia caused by a re-entrant mechanism. They are demonstrated by signal-averaged electrocardiography. The ECG is recorded with an orthogonal system: leads are placed in the fourth intercostal space in both midaxillary lines, on the front (lead V2 position) and back of the chest, and top and bottom of the sternum. Computerized signal averaging and appropriate filtering of a series of QRS complexes eliminate electrical noise, which is random, and the main part of the QRS complex and thereby demonstrate late potentials (Figure 5.11).

Widely used criteria for late potentials are the presence of two of the following three observations:

1. Filtered QRS duration >110 ms
2. Root mean square of last 40 ms of QRS complex <25 ms
3. Duration of terminal portion of QRS complex <40 µV exceeds 32 ms.

Late potentials indicate the presence of the substrate for ventricular tachycardia, i.e. an area of slowed conduction, not that spontaneous ventricular tachycardia will necessarily occur. In patients who present with ventricular tachycardia, late potentials show that the arrhythmia should be inducible at electrophysiological study. Late potentials after myocardial infarction point to a poor prognosis, particularly where there is evidence of extensive myocardial damage.

Prognosis

Ventricular tachycardia that is not due to an acute event such as acute myocardial infarction or drug toxicity is likely to recur.

Ventricular tachycardias vary in their prognosis according to their cause and the resultant symptoms and haemodynamic disturbance, as summarized in Table 5.3.

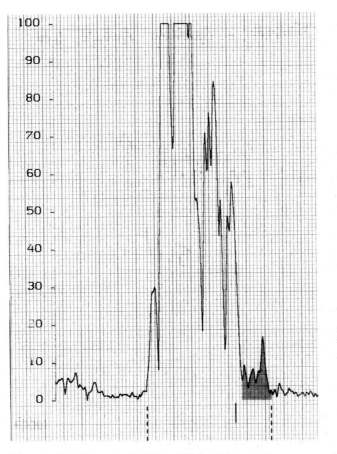

Figure 5.11 Shaded area indicates late potential. Filtered QRS = 167 ms, root mean square of terminal 40 ms = 7 µV and duration of high frequency low amplitude signals in terminal 40 ms = 48 ms

Table 5.3 Factors influencing risk of ventricular tachycardia

	High risk	*Lower risk*
Causes	Ischaemic HOCM* COCM†	Idiopathic RV dysplasia fascicular
Arrhythmia	Arrest/syncope hypotensive sustained inducible	Palpitation non-hypotensive non-sustained non-inducible

* HOCM = hypertrophic cardiomyopathy.
† COCM = dilated cardiomyopathy.

Usually, non-sustained ventricular tachycardia has no prognostic significance. However, in hypertrophic cardiomyopathy it does indicate a significant risk of sudden death.

Treatment

Choice of treatment depends on what symptoms the arrhythmia causes, whether the arrhythmia is likely to recur, and the prognosis.

Termination of tachycardia

Options include cardioversion, drugs, pacing and electrical stimulation.

Cardioversion

If sustained ventricular tachycardia causes cardiac arrest or shock, immediate cardioversion is necessary (see Chapter 13). Cardioversion should also be undertaken if anti-arrhythmic drugs are ineffective, contraindicated or cause haemodynamic deterioration without restoring normal rhythm.

Anti-arrhythmic drugs

Lignocaine is the first-line drug for termination of ventricular tachycardia. Other drugs that are commonly used are mexiletine, disopyramide, sotalol and flecainide. The last three drugs are markedly negatively inotropic and are best avoided in patients with heart failure or in those known to have extensive myocardial damage. In general, no more than two drugs should be given before considering alternative methods of arrhythmia termination.

Amiodarone is a very useful second-line drug. It does not have a significant negative inotropic action and is extremely effective. However, it rarely works 'at the end of a needle' and can take up to 24 hours to act. If ventricular tachycardia keeps recurring it may be worth using amiodarone despite its delayed action, rather than risking the complications associated with other less effective drugs – even if cardioversion or pacing is required while amiodarone is taking effect.

Though verapamil is effective in controlling supraventricular tachycardia it is, with the exception of fascicular and right ventricular outflow tract tachycardia, useless in ventricular tachycardia and may cause severe hypotension. It is dangerous practice to use the drug as a therapeutic test to ascertain the origin of a tachycardia with broad QRS complexes.

Pacing

Pacing can sometimes be successful in terminating ventricular tachycardia (Figure 5.12). It should be considered when drugs are ineffective, when frequently recurrent tachycardia necessitates multiple cardioversions or when a temporary pacing wire is already in place for treatment of a bradycardia.

The usual method is overdrive right ventricular pacing. A burst for a few seconds at a rate 10–30% in excess of that of the tachycardia will often terminate the arrhythmia. However, there is a significant risk of accelerating the tachycardia or precipitating ventricular fibrillation; in which case cardioversion will be necessary.

In patients where there is a high risk should ventricular tachycardia recur, and in whom anti-arrhythmic drugs are ineffective, an automatic implantable cardiovertor defibrillator may be indicated (see below).

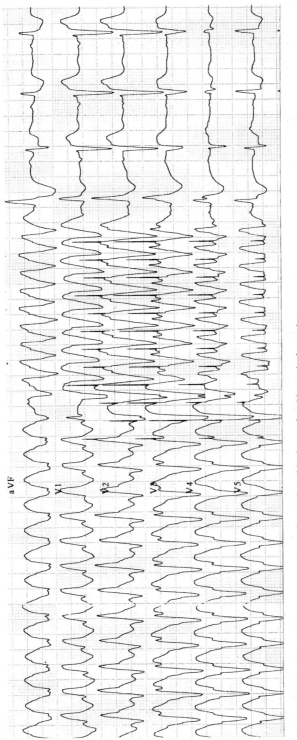

Figure 5.12 Monomorphic ventricular tachycardia terminated by burst of rapid ventricular pacing

Prevention of recurrence of ventricular tachycardia

Intravenous drugs

Blood levels of most anti-arrhythmic drugs fall rapidly after a single bolus. After a bolus injection has restored sinus rhythm it is usual to give a continuous infusion of the drug. This makes sense if ventricular tachycardia is expected to recur within a short period, e.g. after acute myocardial infarction. However, it is pointless to set up an infusion if either the bolus has failed or if the tachycardia is known to occur infrequently.

Oral drugs

Unless ventricular tachycardia occurs during acute myocardial infarction or other acute events, recurrence is likely and long-term therapy is indicated. Therapy is particularly important if the arrhythmia is associated with significant structural heart disease or has caused marked hypotension or shock, since the prognosis without treatment is poor.

Several drugs may be useful: sotalol, disopyramide, flecainide and amiodarone. When ventricular tachycardia has been provoked by exertion, beta-blockers are often effective. Disopyramide, flecainide and beta-blockers may precipitate heart failure in patients with extensive myocardial damage. Amiodarone is the most effective drug but often causes unwanted effects. In patients who are at high risk from further arrhythmias it would seem reasonable to use amiodarone and consider alternatives if major side-effects occur.

Occasionally a single drug will not prevent ventricular tachycardia. If tachycardia is refractory to single drugs given in appropriate dose, it may be necessary to resort to a combination of drugs from different anti-arrhythmic classes, e.g. amiodarone plus mexiletine, amiodarone plus xamoterol or a beta-blocker, or quinidine plus mexiletine (see Chapter 12).

Pacing

Sometimes ventricular tachycardia arises during bradycardia. If the heart rate is low, e.g. <50 beats/minute, the rate should be increased by pacing before drugs are given: often pacing alone will prevent ventricular tachycardia.

Pacing at a rate of 80–90/minute together with drugs may prevent ventricular tachycardia when the rate during sinus rhythm is relatively slow, e.g. 50–70 beats/minute.

Surgery

If ventricular tachycardia is refractory to anti-arrhythmic drugs then surgery should be considered. There are several techniques which involve the excision or isolation of the arrhythmia focus. However, potential candidates for surgery often have impaired myocardial function. Cardiopulmonary bypass surgery carries a substantial risk when myocardial function is poor, since ventriculotomy may worsen function.

Occasionally, life-threatening, resistant ventricular arrhythmias are an indication for cardiac transplantation.

Catheter ablation

Some success has been achieved in preventing ventricular tachycardia by delivering either high-energy direct current shocks or radio-frequency energy via an electrode catheter to the site of origin of tachycardia.

Assessment of efficacy

Whatever treatment is chosen, it is important to ensure it is effective in preventing a recurrence of ventricular tachycardia. If the tachycardia has been frequent then monitoring the electrocardiogram at the bedside or using ambulatory electrocardiography is the best method of assessing efficacy. Where control has been difficult to achieve it may be necessary to accept some ventricular extrasystoles and even short runs of ventricular tachycardia, provided that the rate during tachycardia is considerably slower than before treatment.

If ventricular tachycardia has been infrequent then it is unlikely that ECG monitoring will reflect anti-arrhythmic control. Exercise ECG testing and electrophysiological testing may be helpful.

Most anti-arrhythmic drugs can be pro-arrhythmic. Class Ic drugs (Chapter 12) are the commonest culprits and patients with extensive myocardial damage the most susceptible. If no headway is being made in maintaining normal rhythm or there are new arrhythmias, a pro-arrhythmic effect should be considered.

Polymorphic ventricular tachycardia

Whereas monomorphic ventricular tachycardia consists of a rapid succession of ventricular ectopic beats each with the same configuration, polymorphic ventricular tachycardia is characterized by repeated progressive changes in the QRS complex so the complexes 'twist' about the baseline (Figure 5.13). It may result from acute myocardial infarction and from other causes of myocardial damage. In these situations the QT interval during sinus rhythm is usually normal and the management of the arrhythmia is the same as for monomorphic ventricular tachycardia.

Torsade de pointes tachycardia

This term refers to polymorphic ventricular tachycardia when the QT interval is prolonged during sinus rhythm (Figure 5.14). Often there are prominent U waves. Recognition is important because anti-arrhythmic drugs may aggravate the tachycardia and because correction of its cause should prevent it.

The arrhythmia is caused by bradycardia or by drugs or disorders that lead to abnormal ventricular repolarization (Table 5.4). Usually it is non-sustained and repetitive.

Management

Treatment consists of reversal of the cause where possible, and cardiac pacing.

Anti-arrhythmic drugs should be stopped. Increasing the heart rate to 100 beats/minute by pacing will often prevent the tachycardia while the drug(s) are being excreted or metabolized.

A few patients have a long QT interval even without anti-arrhythmic therapy. In these patients, drugs such as quinidine and disopyramide which can markedly prolong QT interval should not be used, to avoid the risk of torsade de pointes tachycardia.

Table 5.4 Causes of torsade de pointes tachycardia

Bradycardia due to sick sinus syndrome or atrioventricular block
Anti-arrhythmic drugs
Congenital prolongation of the QT interval
Hypokalaemia, hypomagnesaemia
Drugs, e.g. prenylamine, tricyclic antidepressants, erythromycin

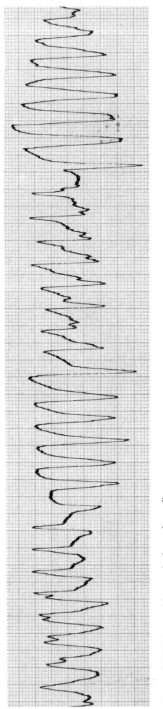

Figure 5.13 Polymorphic ventricular tachycardia

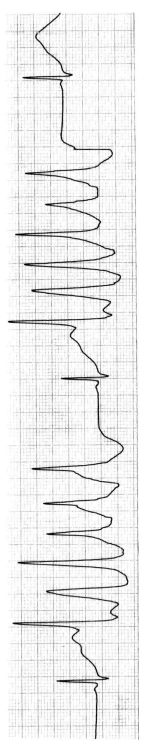

Figure 5.14 Two episodes of torsade de pointes tachycardia during sinus bradycardia: there is marked QT prolongation

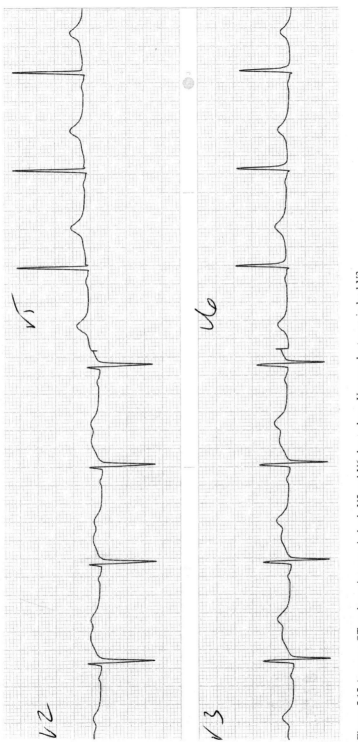

Figure 5.15 Apparent QT prolongation seen in leads V5 and V6 due to large U waves best seen in lead V3

There are reports that intravenous magnesium sulphate may be effective even when serum magnesium is normal.

QT interval

The QT interval is a measure of the duration of ventricular repolarization. It is measured from the onset of the QRS complex to the end of the T wave. Precise measurement is difficult because the timing of these events varies from ECG lead to lead and because it can be difficult to define the point at which the T wave ends and U wave starts (Figure 5.15).

Prolongation of the QT interval suggests either there is uniform prolongation of the process of repolarization throughout the myocardium or that regions of myocardium vary in their rates of repolarization. The latter situation is the one likely to cause ventricular arrhythmias.

The QT interval normally shortens with increasing heart rate, partly due to the increase in rate itself and partly due to the increase in sympathetic nervous system activity associated with sinus tachycardia. When measuring the QT interval it is necessary to correct the measured interval for heart rate. The corrected QT interval (QTc) is usually calculated by dividing the square root of the cycle length into the measured QT interval. The normal QTc does not exceed 0.42 s.

Congenital prolongation of the QT interval

The Romano–Ward syndrome and the Jervel and Lange–Nielson syndrome are two conditions in which there is congenital prolongation of the QT interval and a tendency to ventricular tachycardia, usually polymorphic. The former is due to a dominant gene; the latter is due to a recessive gene and is associated with nerve deafness.

Ventricular tachycardia is usually induced by exertion or emotion as a result of high levels of sympathetic activity and may cause syncope. Sudden death can occur. The disorders are thought to be due to imbalance between left and right sympathetic innervation of the heart. During exercise the QT interval may not shorten and may become prolonged.

Full beta-blockade is often effective. Cardiac pacing in addition to beta-blockers should be considered in those patients with marked bradycardia prior to or because of beta-blockers.

Left cervical sympathectomy is indicated where beta-blockade has failed.

Automatic Implantable Cardiovertor Defibrillator

This is an implantable device which can recognize and automatically terminate ventricular tachycardia or fibrillation by delivering an appropriate electrical therapy: precisely timed pacing stimuli, low energy (0.5–10 J) d.c. shock, i.e. cardioversion, or higher energy (15–35 J) d.c. shock, i.e. defibrillation (Figures 5.16 and 5.17). In addition, the device can act as an ordinary pacemaker to prevent bradycardia.

Because the devices are substantially bigger than pacemakers, implantation in the rectus sheath is usually necessary. Early systems employed epicardial lead and necessitated thoracotomy, but now transvenous leads are widely used.

Many patients with cardiac disease are at risk of sudden death due to ventricular tachycardia or fibrillation and might benefit from the device. However, its benefits have to be weighed against its shortcomings.

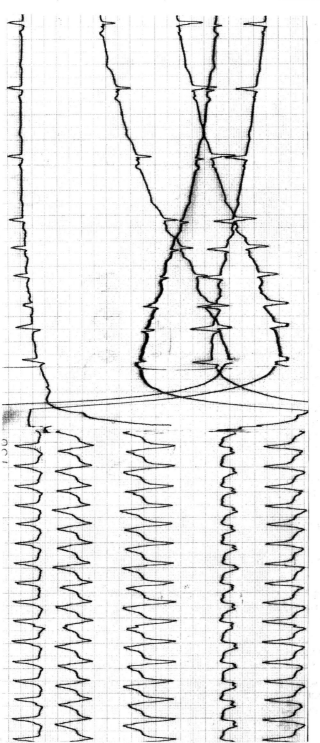

Figure 5.16 Transvenous cardioversion of ventricular tachycardia

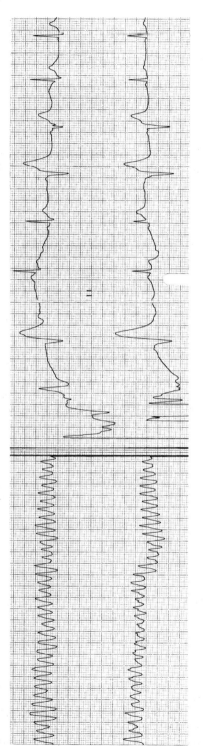

Figure 5.17 Termination of ventricular fibrillation by implanted defibrillator

Indications

The principal indications are for those patients who are at high risk from a recurrence of their arrhythmia:

1. Survivors of sudden cardiac death not caused by acute myocardial infarction or by a correctable cause such as hypokalaemia, particularly if their arrhythmia is inducible at electrophysiological testing in spite of drugs. There is good evidence to show that survival is improved in this group.
2. Patients who have experienced recurrent ventricular tachycardia which has caused syncope or severe hypotension which cannot be prevented by drugs.
3. In some patients, ventricular tachycardia can be terminated by precisely timed ventricular pacing stimuli or by burst pacing, but there is a significant risk that pacing will accelerate the tachycardia or precipitate ventricular fibrillation. The device can be programmed to deliver pacing stimuli and then to deliver a low or high energy shock should pacing be ineffective or cause a more major arrhythmia.

Limitations

The device is not suitable for patients with frequently recurrent or incessant tachycardia since it would be activated too often.

The device may be inappropriately activated. Detection of ventricular tachycardia and fibrillation is based mainly on measurement of ventricular rate. It is recognized that the device may discharge inappropriately in response to a rapid ventricular rate during atrial fibrillation or to non-sustained ventricular tachycardia; discharge of a d.c. shock in a conscious patient results in sudden marked chest discomfort and often causes considerable distress!

The devices do not always reliably recognize ventricular tachycardia or fibrillation and can provide only a limited number (approximately 300) of shocks before having to be replaced.

To lose consciousness from ventricular fibrillation and then be defibrillated is not a pleasant experience for a patient. Ideally, the implantable defibrillator should act as a 'backup' device, only to be used if other anti-arrhythmic measures have failed. On the other hand, anti-arrhythmic drugs such as amiodarone may raise the 'defibrillation threshold' and render the device ineffective.

Currently costs are high. In the UK in 1992, implantation costs are in excess of £15 000.

Complications such as infection, device erosion, lead fracture and psychiatric disturbance are not uncommon.

Future

In the future, a smaller device which requires only transvenous leads, which can accurately detect a major arrhythmia and deliver the appropriate electrical therapy – extrastimuli, micro-shock or if necessary defibrillation – can be expected. If costs decrease and reliability increases, the indications for implantation may extend to all patients considered to be at significant risk of a dangerous ventricular arrhythmia.

Main points

- Monomorphic ventricular tachycardia consists of a rapid, regular succession of ventricular extrasystoles each with the same configuration. Their duration exceeds 0.12 s and is usually greater than 0.14 s.
- The common causes of ventricular tachycardia are myocardial damage from coronary artery disease or from cardiomyopathy.
- Wherever possible, obtain and save a 12-lead ECG during tachycardia.
- The presence of P waves dissociated from ventricular activity or of fusion or capture beats indicates independent atrial activity and confirms ventricular tachycardia.
- If the tachycardia causes shock, prompt cardioversion is indicated.
- Lignocaine is the first-line drug for intravenous use. Generally, no than two drugs should be tried before resorting to amiodarone or non-pharmacological methods of treatment. Verapamil should not be given except for right ventricular outflow tract and fascicular tachycardias.
- It is important to try to ensure that long-term anti-arrhythmic therapy is effective since ventricular tachycardia is often a recurrent problem and may lead to sudden death.
- Accelerated idioventricular rhythm is ventricular tachycardia at a rate less than 120 beats/minute. Treatment is not required.
- Polymorphic tachycardia is characterized by repeated progressive changes in the QRS complex so the complexes appear to 'twist' about the baseline.
- Torsade de pointes tachycardia refers to polymorphic tachycardia when there is QT prolongation during sinus rhythm. Anti-arrhythmic therapy may aggravate the arrhythmia and pacing is often effective.

Supraventricular tachycardias

Main types

Several tachycardias originate from the atria or AV junction and are therefore supraventricular in origin (Table 6.1). They have one thing in common: because they arise from above the level of the bundle branches, they usually result in narrow ventricular complexes. However, it is important to appreciate there are important differences in mechanism, ECG characteristic and treatment. It is necessary to identify the type of tachycardia and not merely treat all tachycardias with narrow QRS complexes as 'supraventricular tachycardia'.

Table 6.1 Supraventricular tachycardias

1. Atrial fibrillation
2. Atrial flutter
3. Atrial tachycardia
4. Atrioventricular re-entrant tachycardia
5. Atrioventricular nodal re-entrant
   tachycardia
6. Sinus tachycardia (see Chapter 1)

Atrial origin versus atrioventricular re-entry

There are two main types of supraventricular tachycardias.

First, there are the atrioventricular re-entrant tachycardias. An additional connection between atria and ventricles is present so an impulse can repeatedly pass between atria and ventricles along a circuit consisting of the AV junction and the additional AV connection.

The second group comprises those caused by rapid atrial activity, i.e. atrial tachycardia, flutter and fibrillation. The mechanism responsible for the tachycardia is confined to the atria. In contrast to the first group, the AV node is not an integral part of the tachycardia mechanism but merely transmits some or all the atrial impulses to the ventricles.

Atrioventricular re-entrant tachycardias

Mechanism

In most cases the heart is structurally normal, i.e. there is no valve, myocardial or coronary disease.

The arrhythmia is caused by the repeated circulation of an impulse between atria and ventricles. It can only occur if there are two – rather than the usual one – connections between atria and ventricles. The impulse is usually conducted from atria to ventricles by the AV junction and then re-enters the atria via the additional connection (Figure 6.1). The additional connection is either an accessory AV pathway which bypasses the AV node (Wolff–Parkinson–White syndrome, Chapter 7) or is actually part of, but functionally separate from, the AV node.

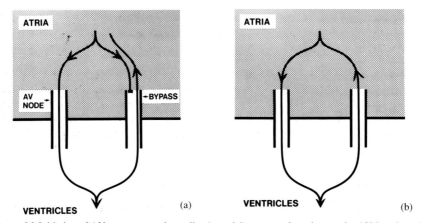

Figure 6.1 Initiation of AV re-entrant tachycardia. An atrial extrasystole arrives at the AV junction while the bypass tract is still refractory to excitation. The extrasystole is therefore only conducted to the ventricles via the AV node. By the time the extrasystole has traversed the AV node and reached the ventricles, the bypass tract has recovered and can conduct the impulse back to the atria (a) thereby initiating the re-entrant mechanism (b)

A re-entrant tachycardia involving an accessory AV pathway is termed an AV re-entrant tachycardia while a tachycardia due to dual AV nodal pathways is termed an AV nodal re-entrant tachycardia. With the latter, conduction from atria to ventricles is usually via a relatively slowly conducting AV nodal pathway while ventriculo-atrial conduction is via a fast AV nodal tract.

ECG characteristics

The rhythm is regular and usually the QRS complexes are narrow (Figure 6.2). Occasionally pre-existing bundle branch block or bundle branch block caused by the tachycardia will lead to broad ventricular complexes (Figure 6.3).

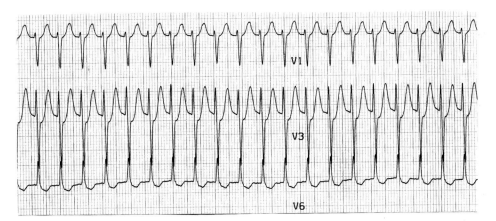

Figure 6.2 AV re-entrant tachycardia. A regular tachycardia with narrow ventricular complexes

The rate during tachycardia can range from 130 to 250 beats/minute and is influenced by the sympathetic nervous system. For example, sympathetic activity and consequently the speed of AV nodal conduction increase on standing up so the tachycardia becomes faster.

Clearly, normal P waves will not occur during this arrhythmia. Since the circulating impulse re-enters the atria after ventricular activation, each QRS complex will be followed by an inverted P wave, though this wave is not always detectable. If the atrial rate exceeds the ventricular rate, whether spontaneously or due to a drug or manoeuvre which slows AV node conduction, then the rhythm is not atrioventricular re-entrant tachycardia: it is probably atrial tachycardia or flutter.

Timing of atrial activity

The timing of atrial activity during tachycardia, if identifiable, may indicate whether the tachycardia is due to an accessory AV pathway, i.e. AV re-entry, or due to an additional AV nodal connection, i.e. AV nodal re-entry.

With AV nodal re-entrant tachycardia, an inverted P wave immediately follows or is superimposed on the QRS complex because the re-entrant circuit is small (Figures 6.4 and 6.5). In contrast, the length of the re-entrant circuit is greater in the Wolff–Parkinson–White syndrome because the accessory AV pathway is some distance from the AV junction. It therefore takes longer for an impulse to circulate and re-enter the atria. Hence the inverted P wave occurs roughly halfway between QRS complexes (Figure 6.6).

ST segment and T wave changes can be caused by the tachycardia and persist for some time after its cessation: they are of no diagnostic significance.

The ECG during sinus rhythm is usually normal unless there is pre-excitation (Chapter 7).

Clinical features

The arrhythmia is common. Attacks may start in infancy, childhood or adult life and often recur. The duration and frequency of attacks varies from patient to patient. They may last

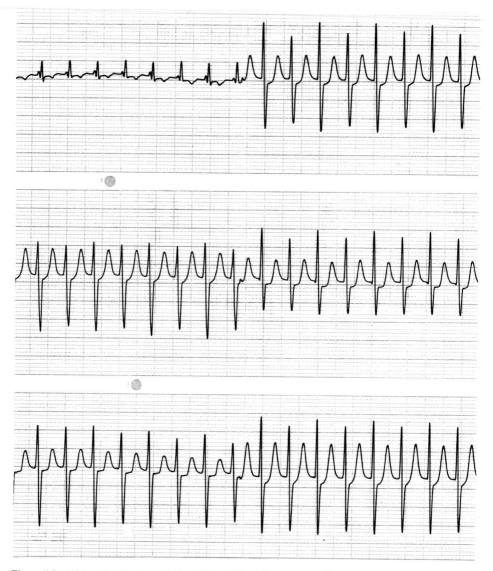

Figure 6.3a AV re-entrant tachycardia, leads V1 to V6, with narrow complexes.

for a few minutes or for many hours, and may recur several times per day or be separated by many months.

In some patients, attacks are precipitated by exertion. In most, episodes can occur at rest or on exertion and can be brought on by trivial activities such as bending down.

The main symptom is rapid and often distressing palpitation of sudden onset. Faintness, syncope, polyuria and chest pain may occur.

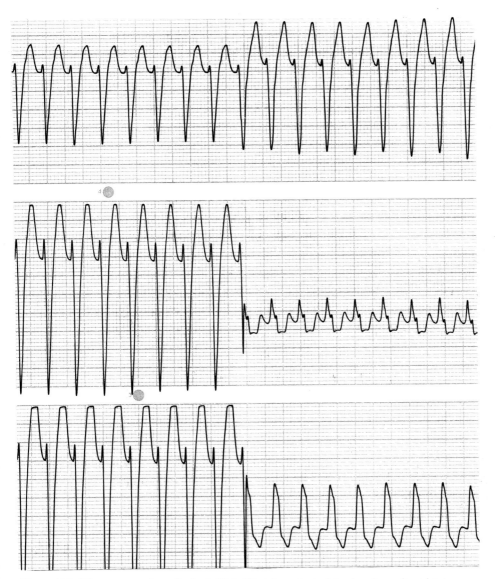

Figure 6.3b AV re-entrant tachycardia, leads V1 to V6. A few minutes later, broad complexes have developed due to functional left bundle branch block

Treatment

The patient should be reassured that the tachycardia is not dangerous and that it is due to an electrical rather than structural cardiac abnormality: patients often fear the arrhythmia is due to coronary disease and that they are at risk from a heart attack.

Treatment is unnecessary for short episodes of tachycardia which do not cause distress.

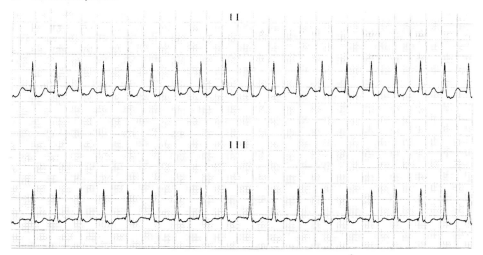

Figure 6.4 AV nodal re-entrant tachycardia. A small P wave immediately follows each QRS complex

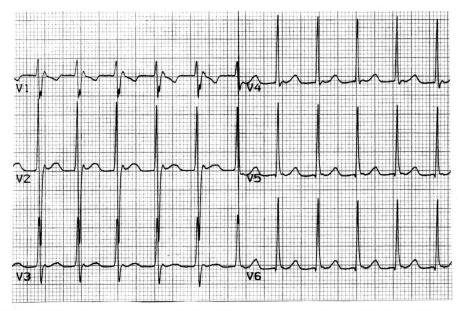

Figure 6.5 AV nodal re-entrant tachycardia. A small P wave can be seen after each QRS. In leads V1 and V2 it could be mistaken for a secondary R wave

The purpose of treatment may be to terminate or to prevent recurrence of the arrhythmia (Table 6.3).

Vagal stimulation

The first approach to termination is vagal stimulation. An increase in vagal tone may temporarily slow conduction through the AV node and thereby interrupt the tachycardia circuit.

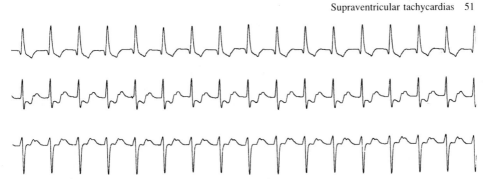

Figure 6.6 AV re-entrant tachycardia (leads I, II, III). There is a P wave after each QRS complex which is superimposed on the T wave, resulting in its pointed appearance. An inverted P wave in lead I suggests a left-sided accessory pathway

Table 6.2 The characteristics of AV re-entrant tachycardias

QRS complexes:
  regular
  rate 130–250 beats/minute
  usually narrow

P waves:
  inverted, after each QRS complex
  often concealed by superimposed terminal portion of ventricular complex

Table 6.3 Summary of treatments for AV re-entrant tachycardia

Termination:
  vagal stimulation
  intravenous drugs, e.g. adenosine, verapamil
  cardioversion
  pacing (overdrive, underdrive or programmed stimulation)

Prevention:
  drugs, e.g. sotalol, flecainide
  ablation of accessory connection
  ablation or modification of AV node

The Valsalva manoeuvre and carotid sinus massage are the best methods. The former is performed by attempting to forcefully expire for 10–15 s while the nose and mouth are sealed. Carotid massage is performed by firm digital pressure over one carotid artery at the level of the upper border of the thyroid cartilage for 5 s.

Eyeball pressure is widely quoted as a method for vagal stimulation but is very painful and should not be used.

Intravenous drugs

If vagal stimulation fails, the tachycardia can almost certainly be terminated by an intravenous injection of one of several drugs. Verapamil has been widely used but adenosine, recently introduced, is now the treatment of choice.

Adenosine

Adenosine is a potent blocker of AV nodal conduction which has an extremely short duration of action of 20–30 s. It is very effective in terminating AV re-entrant tachycardias (Figure 6.7).

It should be given as a rapid (2 s) intravenous bolus, followed by a saline flush. The initial dose in adults and in children is 3 mg and 0.05 mg/kg, respectively. If ineffective, further dosages of 6 mg (0.10 mg/kg) and, if necessary, 12 mg can be given after 1-minute intervals up to a maximum of 12 mg (0.25 mg/kg).

Many patients will experience chest tightness, dyspnoea and flushing but the symptoms last less than 60 s. There may be complete AV block for a few seconds following termination of the tachycardia. A few ventricular ectopic beats may also occur. The drug does not have a negative inotropic action.

Verapamil

Intravenous verapamil (5–10 mg over 30–60 s) will usually restore sinus rhythm within a couple of minutes.

Verapamil must not be used if the patient has recently received an oral or intravenous beta-blocking drug (see Chapter 12).

Other drugs

Drugs such as sotalol, disopyramide and flecainide may also be effective (see Chapter 12).

Electrical methods

Pacing

Various pacing methods may terminate AV re-entrant tachycardias. The simplest is pacing the right atrium at a rate 20–30% faster than the tachycardia (overdrive pacing). On abrupt termination of pacing, sinus rhythm will often return: if unsuccessful, pacing should be repeated (Figure 6.8). There is a small risk of precipitating atrial fibrillation which usually will not last for many minutes before sinus rhythm is restored. However, in patients with Wolff–Parkinson–White syndrome atrial fibrillation might lead to a very fast ventricular response (see Chapter 7).

More sophisticated methods require a programmable pacemaker which allows the introduction of precisely timed extrastimuli (Figure 6.9). These methods can be used on a long-term basis by implanting a pacemaker (Figure 6.10). An intracardiac electrophysiological study is necessary to assess suitability of long-term pacing.

Cardioversion

If drugs are ineffective or if clinical circumstances necessitate an immediate return to sinus rhythm, cardioversion should be carried out (see Chapter 13).

Prevention

There are two main approaches: drug therapy; or ablation or modification of part of the re-entry circuit.

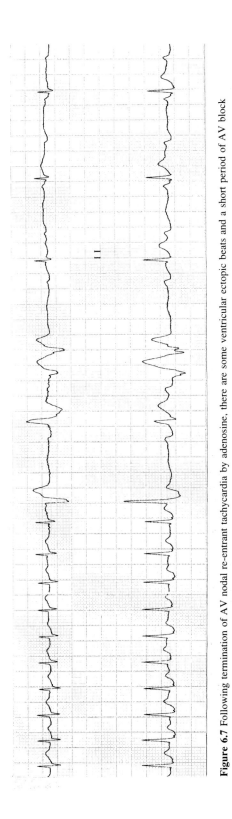

Figure 6.7 Following termination of AV nodal re-entrant tachycardia by adenosine, there are some ventricular ectopic beats and a short period of AV block

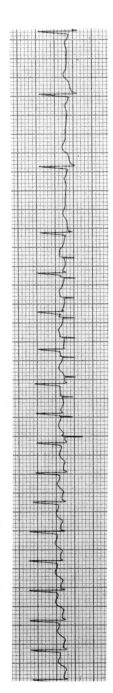
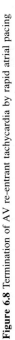

Figure 6.8 Termination of AV re-entrant tachycardia by rapid atrial pacing

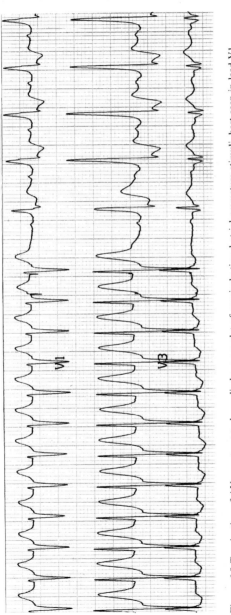

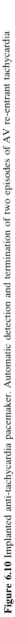

Figure 6.9 Termination of AV re-entrant tachycardia by a couplet of precisely timed atrial premature stimuli, best seen in lead V1, revealing Wolff–Parkinson–White syndrome on return to sinus rhythm

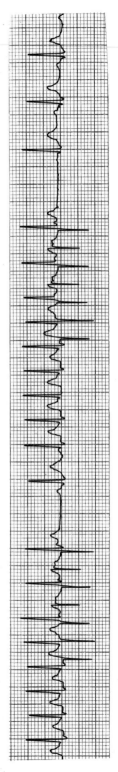

Figure 6.10 Implanted anti-tachycardia pacemaker. Automatic detection and termination of two episodes of AV re-entrant tachycardia

Drugs

Selection of a drug which is both effective and well tolerated is often a process of trial and error. The patient should keep a record of the date and duration of any attacks so that the effect of therapy can be assessed.

Sotalol (160–320 mg daily) is a good first-line drug (see Chapter 12). Flecainide and disopyramide are alternatives.

Amiodarone is likely to be effective where other drugs have failed, but should be reserved for refractory cases where the need for tachycardia control outweighs the drug's possible unwanted effects and non-pharmacological methods (see below) cannot be used.

Ablation

In patients with AV re-entrant tachycardia, ablation of the accessory AV pathway will prevent the arrhythmia. In the past this could only be achieved by surgery. Now percutaneous ablation is possible. Radiofrequency energy can be delivered to the bypass tract by an electrode advanced to the heart via a vein or artery. A detailed intracardiac electrophysiological study is required to locate the additional AV connection.

AV nodal re-entrant tachycardia can be prevented by delivery of radiofrequency energy to the region of the AV node. Tracts of fast and slow conduction can be identified and one or other ablated.

Re-entrant tachycardia can also be prevented by creation of complete AV block using either radiofrequency or direct current electrical energy but this necessitates implantation of a rate-responsive pacemaker (Figure 6.11).

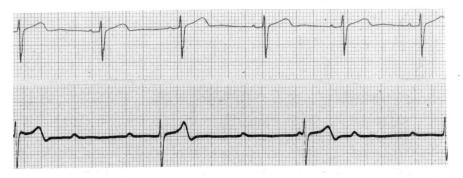

Figure 6.11 Patient with paroxysmal supraventricular tachycardia before (upper trace) and after (lower trace) transvenous AV nodal ablation

Atrial arrhythmias

This group consists of those supraventricular arrhythmias caused by rapid atrial activity, i.e. atrial tachycardia, flutter and fibrillation. In contrast to the AV re-entrant tachycardias, the mechanism responsible for the tachycardia is confined to the atria. The AV node merely transmits some or all the atrial impulses to the ventricles. Drugs that impair AV nodal conduction cannot be expected to restore normal rhythm, though they should slow the ventricular rate.

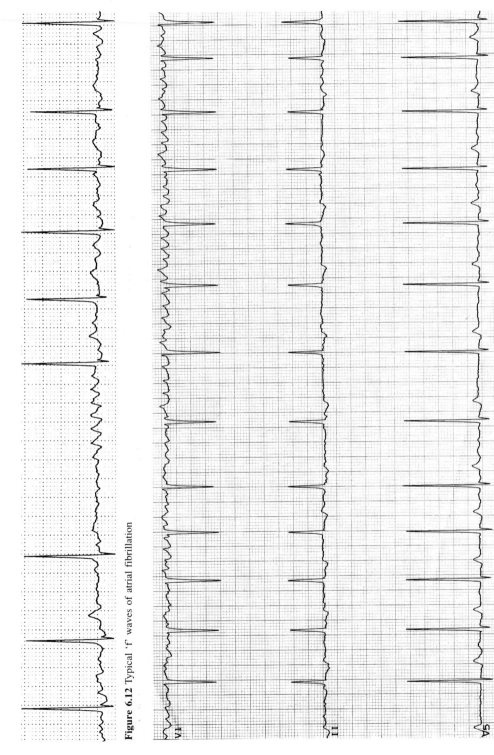

Figure 6.12 Typical 'f' waves of atrial fibrillation

Figure 6.13 Atrial fibrillation. 'f' waves appear coarse in V1, fine in II and are not seen in V5. There is a totally irregular ventricular rhythm

Atrial fibrillation

During atrial fibrillation, the atria discharge at a rate between 350 and 600/minute.

ECG characteristics

Atrial activity
The rapid and chaotic atrial activity during atrial fibrillation results in small, irregular 'f' waves at a rate of 350–600/minute. The amplitude of 'f' waves varies from ECG lead to lead. In some leads, 'f' waves may not be apparent whereas in other leads, especially lead V1, the waves may appear so coarse that atrial flutter is suspected (Figures 6.12 and 6.13).

Atrioventricular conduction
Fortunately, the atrioventricular node cannot conduct every atrial impulse to the ventricles. Some are totally blocked. Others only partially penetrate the atrioventricular node. They will not therefore activate the ventricles but may block or delay succeeding impulses. This process of 'concealed conduction' is responsible for the totally irregular ventricular rhythm during atrial fibrillation which is the hallmark of this arrhythmia.

In the absence of P waves, even if 'f' waves are not seen, a totally irregular ventricular rhythm is diagnostic of atrial fibrillation. Atrial fibrillation with a rapid ventricular rhythm is often misdiagnosed. If the characteristic irregular rhythm is remembered, this mistake will not be made (Figure 6.14). If, however, there is complete atrioventricular block, ventricular activity will, of course, be slow and regular (Figure 6.15).

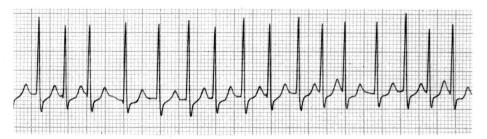

Figure 6.14 Atrial fibrillation with rapid ventricular response

The ventricular rate during atrial fibrillation is dependent on the conducting ability of the AV node which is itself influenced by the autonomic system. Atrioventricular conduction will be enhanced by sympathetic nervous system activity and depressed by high vagal tone. In patients with normal atrioventricular conduction, the ventricular rate ranges from 100 to 180 beats/minute.

Intraventricular conduction
Ventricular complexes during atrial fibrillation are of normal duration unless there is established bundle branch block, Wolff–Parkinson–White syndrome or aberrant intraventricular conduction. Aberrant conduction is the result of unequal recovery periods of the bundle branches. An early atrial impulse may reach the ventricles when one bundle branch is refractory but the other is capable of conduction. The resultant ventricular complex will have a bundle branch block configuration. Because the right bundle usually

has the longer refractory period, aberrant conduction commonly leads to right bundle branch block. The duration of the refractory period is related to the preceding cycle length. Thus, aberration is likely to occur when a short cycle succeeds a long cycle (Figure 6.16).

Initiation
Atrial fibrillation is usually initiated by an atrial extrasystole (Figure 6.17). Sometimes atrial flutter or atrioventricular re-entrant tachycardia degenerate into atrial fibrillation.

Table 6.4 Characteristics of atrial fibrillation

Ventricular activity:
  totally irregular

Atrial activity:
  P waves absent
  'f' waves to be seen in at least some leads

Causes

The main causes are coronary, hypertensive and rheumatic heart diseases, hyperthyroidism, sick sinus syndrome, dilated cardiomyopathy, hypertrophic cardiomyopathy, openheart surgery, thoracotomy, chronic obstructive airways disease, acute or chronic alcohol abuse, and constrictive pericarditis. In a substantial proportion of cases, atrial fibrillation is idiopathic, i.e. there is no demonstrable cause.

Coronary heart disease *per se* does not cause atrial fibrillation. However, the arrhythmia often results from myocardial infarction, both acutely and in the long term, and is an indicator of extensive myocardial damage.

A cause for atrial fibrillation should always be sought. Many of the causes can be identified or excluded by clinical examination, electrocardiography and echocardiography. Measurement of serum thyroxine is often necessary to exclude hyperthyroidism. Ambulatory electrocardiography may be required where sick sinus syndrome is a possibility.

Prevalence

Atrial fibrillation is common. Prevalence increases with age. In a survey of male civil servants in the UK, atrial fibrillation was found in 0.16, 0.37 and 1.13% of those aged 40–49, 50–59 and 60–64 years, respectively. 3.7% of patients over 65 years in a British general practice were found to have the arrhythmia.

Prognosis

One of the major determinants of prognosis is the presence or absence of organic heart disease. For example, in patients with coronary artery disease, because atrial fibrillation is usually a result of extensive myocardial damage, it indicates a poor prognosis. Idiopathic atrial fibrillation has a very good prognosis.

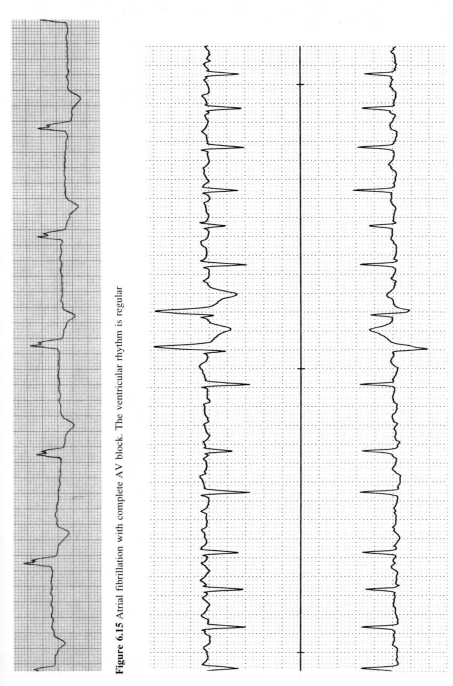

Figure 6.15 Atrial fibrillation with complete AV block. The ventricular rhythm is regular

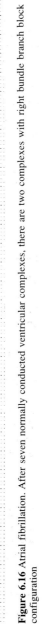

Figure 6.16 Atrial fibrillation. After seven normally conducted ventricular complexes, there are two complexes with right bundle branch block configuration

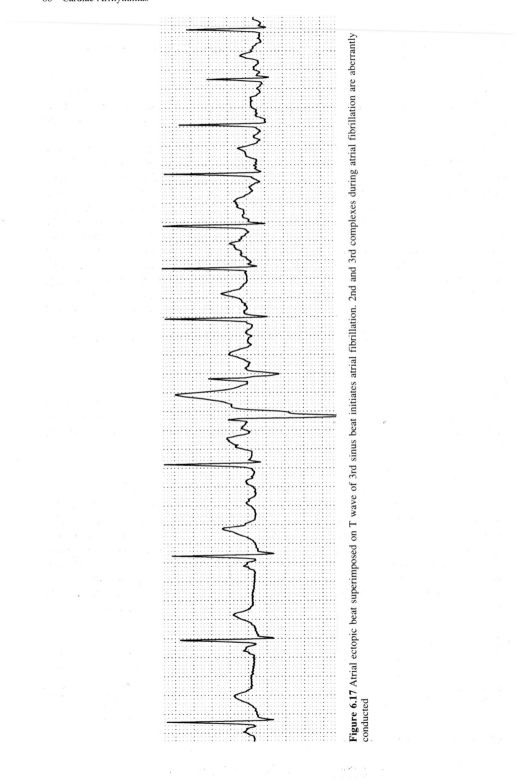

Figure 6.17 Atrial ectopic beat superimposed on T wave of 3rd sinus beat initiates atrial fibrillation. 2nd and 3rd complexes during atrial fibrillation are aberrantly conducted

Systemic embolism

During atrial fibrillation, stasis of blood in the left atrium can lead to thrombus formation and systemic embolism. Of particular concern is the risk of stroke.

Atrial fibrillation caused by rheumatic mitral valve disease is associated with a very high (fifteen-fold) risk of systemic embolism. 'Non-rheumatic' causes of atrial fibrillation lead to a moderate (five-fold) risk of embolism, while the risk is very low in idiopathic atrial fibrillation. The risk of embolism in non-rheumatic atrial fibrillation increases with age: it is small in those less than 60 years.

Oral anticoagulants markedly reduce the risk of embolism and there is evidence to show that aspirin may also be effective. Whereas anticoagulation is strongly indicated in rheumatic atrial fibrillation to reduce the very high risk of embolism, its role in other groups of patients is less clear. Undoubtedly warfarin reduces the incidence of stroke in patients with non-rheumatic atrial fibrillation. However, those who are at risk are mainly elderly. The reduction in risk that warfarin will effect has to be weighed against the hazards of anticoagulant therapy in the elderly, the inconvenience of periodic blood tests and, in view of the prevalence of atrial fibrillation in older age groups, the daunting prospect of anticoagulating at least 2% of the population over 60 years of age. Based on current information, those with non-rheumatic atrial fibrillation who are at high risk (e.g. history of embolism, over 60 years of age, evidence of coronary disease or myocardial dysfunction) who can cope with and have no contraindications to anticoagulation, should receive warfarin.

Aspirin is a more convenient alternative to warfarin for many patients but it remains to be seen whether it is as effective.

Idiopathic atrial fibrillation

Idiopathic or 'lone' atrial fibrillation is a common problem. While the prognosis is good and the risk of systemic embolism is low, lone atrial fibrillation can cause very troublesome symptoms and great anxiety. Like secondary atrial fibrillation, it may be paroxysmal or, less commonly, persistent.

Paroxysmal lone atrial fibrillation

Some patients will experience only a single or a very occasional episode. Others will experience frequent recurrences; perhaps several times in a day. Paroxysms may last for many hours or stop after only a few seconds (Figure 6.18). Some patients will suffer major symptoms: syncope or near-syncope, particularly at the onset of the arrhythmia; distressing palpitation; angina, even in the absence of coronary artery disease; dyspnoea; fatigue and polyuria. Others, including some with frequent attacks and rapid ventricular rates, will be asymptomatic or merely aware of but not distressed by palpitation.

In a minority of patients there will be an identifiable precipitating event such as exercise, vomiting, overindulgence in alcohol, or fatigue. One form of paroxysmal lone

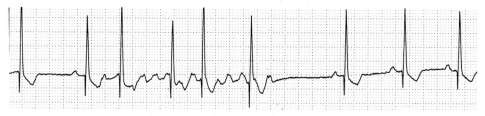

Figure 6.18 A brief episode of atrial fibrillation

atrial fibrillation has been attributed to high vagal activity: the arrhythmia always starts at rest, during bradycardia, and can be initiated by manoeuvres that increase vagal tone.

Treatment

Choice of treatment depends on whether the purpose is to control the ventricular response to atrial fibrillation or to maintain sinus rhythm: a decision which will be influenced by the cause and duration of the arrhythmia.

Treatment of persistent atrial fibrillation is usually aimed at preventing a fast ventricular rate by a drug or drugs which depress atrioventricular nodal conduction. Drugs frequently effect a return to sinus rhythm when the arrhythmia is of recent onset but are otherwise rarely successful. Though cardioversion can usually restore sinus rhythm, atrial fibrillation often recurs.

In paroxysmal atrial fibrillation, oral anti-arrhythmic drugs will often prevent a recurrence.

Control of ventricular response to atrial fibrillation

Digoxin   Oral digoxin provides effective long-term control of persistent atrial fibrillation in many patients and remains the drug of first choice. It has the advantages that it has a long duration of action and is not negatively inotropic. However, digoxin sometimes fails to control the heart rate at rest and is often ineffective at controlling the rate during exertion in spite of high serum concentrations.

Calcium antagonists   Intravenous verapamil quickly and effectively depresses atrioventricular conduction and will thereby control a rapid ventricular response to atrial fibrillation within a few minutes. However, it is unlikely to restore sinus rhythm.

When digoxin alone is inadequate, the addition of oral verapamil (40–80 mg tds) is extremely effective in controlling the ventricular rate during atrial fibrillation, both at rest and on exertion. Verapamil increases serum digoxin concentrations but this mechanism is not thought to be responsible for its beneficial effect. Verapamil alone may be effective but is not superior to digoxin.

Diltiazem has similar actions to verapamil.

Beta-blockers   Beta-blocking drugs will also slow the heart rate during atrial fibrillation in digitalized patients but may be contraindicated if myocardial function is impaired.

Restoration of sinus rhythm

Anti-arrhythmic drugs   Oral quinidine, intravenous flecainide, propafenone and sotalol often restore normal rhythm, provided that atrial fibrillation is of recent onset.

Cardioversion   Sinus rhythm can be restored by cardioversion in most patients with atrial fibrillation. However, the arrhythmia frequently returns. Only a minority of patients will remain in normal rhythm in the long term.

Successful cardioversion of atrial fibrillation may require a high energy (300 J) shock. Several drugs such as quinidine, disopyramide, flecainide, sotalol and amiodarone reduce the relapse rate after cardioversion.

While cardioversion only leads to long-term sinus rhythm in a minority of patients, an attempt at restoring sinus rhythm should be considered in those patients with recent atrial fibrillation where no cause has been identified or in whom the disorder which has caused the arrhythmia has resolved or is self-limiting. If there is a recurrence, a further attempt at cardioversion, after initiation of anti-arrhythmic therapy, should only be undertaken in those with troublesome symptoms attributable to the arrhythmia.

Contraindications to cardioversion include presence of atrial fibrillation for more than 12 months and a slow ventricular response in the absence of anti-arrhythmic drugs.

Prevention of recurrence of paroxysmal atrial fibrillation

Several anti-arrhythmic agents can prevent paroxysmal atrial fibrillation. Trial and error is often necessary to find a drug which is both effective and well tolerated.

Sotalol will often prevent a recurrence of paroxysmal atrial fibrillation. Flecainide, disopyramide and propafenone may also be effective.

Quinidine can prevent paroxysmal atrial fibrillation. However, a recent meta-analysis of studies of the efficacy of quinidine in preventing recurrence of atrial fibrillation, found that the drug's use was associated with a significant increase in mortality, presumably due to a pro-arrhythmic effect.

Digoxin shortens the atrial refractory period and may thereby increase the tendency to atrial fibrillation. There is no evidence that it prevents the arrhythmia or slows the ventricular rate during an acute episode.

'Refractory' atrial fibrillation

Amiodarone is a very potent anti-arrhythmic drug which will often maintain sinus rhythm or at least control the ventricular response to atrial fibrillation when other drugs have failed. However, in view of the high incidence of major unwanted effects, the drug should be reserved for patients in whom other drugs have failed and for patients in whom the risk of side-effects in the long term may not be a major consideration because their prognosis is poor, e.g. the elderly and those with severe myocardial damage.

In patients in whom anti-arrhythmic drugs are ineffective or cannot be tolerated, transvenous ablation of the atrioventricular junction should be considered.

Atrial flutter

In atrial flutter the atria discharge at a rate between 250 and 350/minute. In most cases, the atrial rate is close to 300/minute. Atrial flutter is due to a re-entrant circuit within the atria. In the common form of atrial flutter, the circuit lies within the right atrium: an impulse circulates in an inferior direction along the lateral border of the right atrium and returns in a superior direction along the inter-atrial septum.

ECG characteristics

Atrial flutter may be paroxysmal or sustained. It is usually initiated by an atrial extrasystole. It may degenerate into atrial fibrillation.

Atrial activity

During atrial flutter, the atria discharge regularly at a rate of approximately 300 beats/minute. In many leads there will be no isoelectric line between atrial deflections or 'F' waves, leading to the characteristic sawtooth appearance which is usually best seen in leads II,III and AVF. However, in some leads, especially lead V1, atrial activity will be seen in the form of discrete waves (Figure 6.19). Usually, F waves are negative in leads II, III and AVF.

Rapid ventricular activity may sometimes obscure the typical atrial waveform: atrial activity is most likely to be discernible in lead V1.

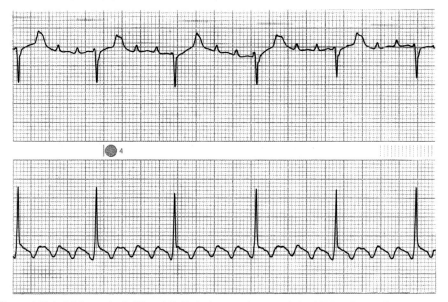

Figure 6.19 Atrial flutter, leads V1 and II. Typical sawtooth pattern in lead II but discrete F waves in lead V1

Atrioventricular conduction

As with atrial fibrillation, the ventricular response to atrial flutter is determined by the conducting ability of the atrioventricular junction. Most commonly, alternate 'F' waves are conducted to the ventricles with a resultant ventricular rate of close to 150 beats/minute (Figure 6.20). Drugs or impaired atrioventricular nodal function may lead to a

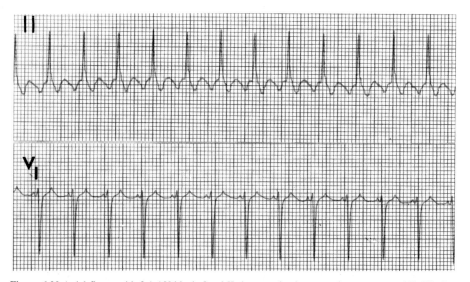

Figure 6.20 Atrial flutter with 2:1 AV block. Lead II shows a classic sawtooth appearance while V1 shows discrete atrial waves. In V1 each QRS complex is immediately preceded by an F wave and is followed by an F wave which is superimposed on the T wave

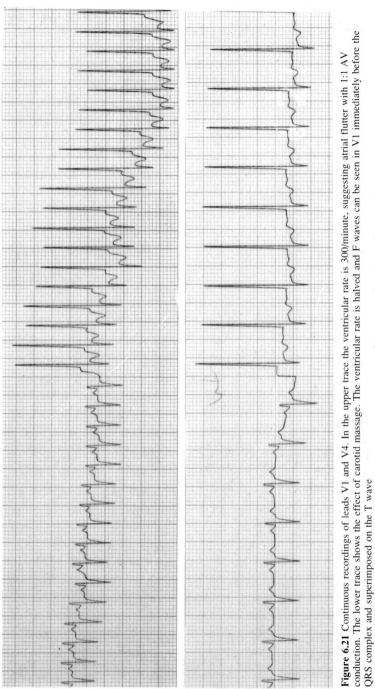

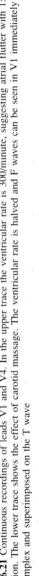

Figure 6.21 Continuous recordings of leads V1 and V4. In the upper trace the ventricular rate is 300/minute, suggesting atrial flutter with 1:1 AV conduction. The lower trace shows the effect of carotid massage. The ventricular rate is halved and F waves can be seen in V1 immediately before the QRS complex and superimposed on the T wave

higher degree of atrioventricular block. High levels of sympathetic nervous system activity, as may occur during exercise, may enhance atrioventricular nodal conduction and result in 1:1 conduction and a ventricular rate of approximately 300 beats/minute (Figure 6.21).

With high degrees of atrioventricular block, atrial activity is clearly discernible and the arrhythmia is easy to diagnose (Figure 6.22). However, during a rapid ventricular response, ventricular T waves may be superimposed on alternate 'F' waves and may obscure the characteristic atrial activity: sinus tachycardia may be mistakenly diagnosed (Figure 6.23). Atrial flutter should be suspected if the heart rate is 150 beats/minute at rest. Carotid sinus massage or adenosine can transiently impair atrioventricular conduction and aid diagnosis (Figure 6.24).

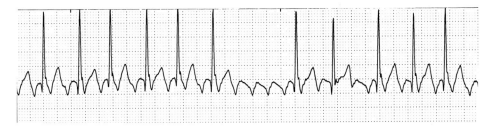

Figure 6.22 Atrial flutter only clearly seen during transient increase in AV block

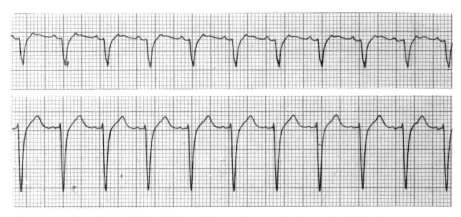

Figure 6.23 Atrial flutter. F waves only clearly seen during transient increase in AV block

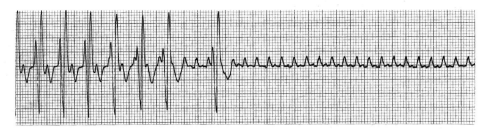

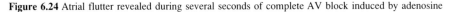

Figure 6.24 Atrial flutter revealed during several seconds of complete AV block induced by adenosine

Intraventricular conduction
Ventricular complexes will be normal in duration unless there is bundle branch block, ventricular pre-excitation or aberrant intraventricular conduction.

Table 6.5   Characteristics of atrial flutter

Atrial activity:
    'F' waves at rate of 300 beats/minute
    may have 'sawtooth' appearance in some leads
    discrete atrial waves may be seen in other leads
Ventricular activity:
    rarely, 1:1 AV conduction resulting in ventricular rate of 300 beats/minute
    usually, 2:1 or higher degrees of AV block

Causes

Atrial flutter has similar aetiologies to atrial fibrillation, though idiopathic atrial flutter is unusual.

Prevalence

Atrial flutter is much less common than atrial fibrillation.

Treatment

Attempts to control a rapid ventricular response to atrial flutter by drugs are often unsuccessful. Where possible, the aim should be to restore and maintain sinus rhythm.

Restoration of normal rhythm

Cardioversion   Sustained atrial flutter can usually be terminated with a low energy d.c. shock, e.g. 25–50 J. If necessary higher energy levels should be used.

Anti-arrhythmic drugs   Drugs such as sotalol, flecainide, disopyramide and propafenone are often effective in terminating atrial flutter. However, it should be borne in mind that under certain circumstances these drugs, if unsuccessful in restoring sinus rhythm, may possibly lead to higher ventricular rates. First, some drugs, particularly disopyramide and quinidine, have a vagolytic effect which might enhance conduction through the atrioventricular node. Secondly, drugs often slow the atrial rate facilitating a reduction in the atrioventricular conduction ratio.

Rapid atrial pacing   Rapid atrial pacing at a rate approximately 10–25% in excess of the atrial rate (not the ventricular rate) for 30–60 s will often restore sinus rhythm. Atrial fibrillation may sometimes be precipitated but usually sinus rhythm will return within a few hours. Pacing is generally carried out transvenously. Stimulation of the posterior septal area of the right atrium is more likely to lead to successful termination of the arrhythmia. The transoesophageal approach is favoured by some. It is important to ensure that pacing stimuli do capture the atria: capture is usually reflected in a change in the ventricular rate.

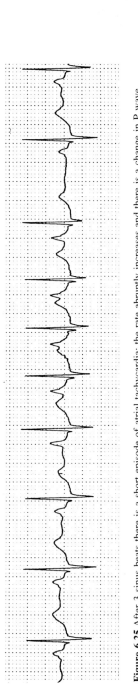

Figure 6.25 After 3 sinus beats there is a short episode of atrial tachycardia: the rate abruptly increases and there is a change in P wave morphology

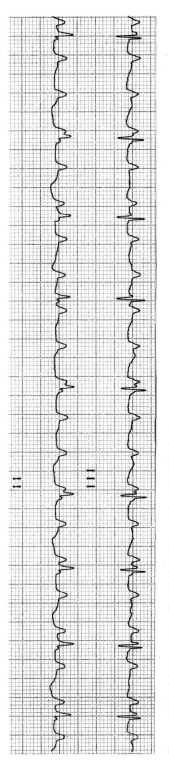

Figure 6.26 Atrial tachycardia with AV block. The atrial rate is 150/minute

Control of ventricular response

If normal rhythm cannot be restored or maintained, atrioventricular nodal blocking drugs may be required to control a rapid ventricular response to atrial flutter. Intravenous verapamil will promptly slow the ventricular rate during atrial flutter. Oral digoxin and/or a calcium antagonist or beta-blocking drug can be employed as with atrial fibrillation.

Maintenance of sinus rhythm

Drugs which may prevent a recurrence of atrial fibrillation, as discussed above, are equally effective in preventing recurrence of atrial flutter.

'Refractory' atrial flutter

Amiodarone can be very effective in maintaining sinus rhythm when other drugs have failed. Even if atrial flutter persists, the drug's actions in both slowing the atrial rate and depressing atrioventricular conduction can lead to a substantial slowing of the ventricular rate.

Transvenous ablation of the atrioventricular junction will achieve control of the ventricular rate.

Atrial tachycardia

The main difference between atrial tachycardia and flutter is that in the former the atrial rate is slower, being between 120 and 250/minute. Again, sometimes the AV node can conduct all atrial impulses but often there is a degree of AV block. (With fairly high grades of AV block, because the atrial rate is relatively slow, the rhythm may be misdiagnosed as complete heart block and an inappropriate request made for cardiac pacing.)

ECG characteristics

Because the atrial rate is slower, there is no sawtooth appearance to the baseline. Abnormally shaped P waves are inscribed at a regular rate (Figures 6.25 and 6.26). Usually, the ventricular complexes will be narrow unless there is pre-existent bundle branch block or phasic aberrant intraventricular conduction.

Atrial tachycardia with 1:1 AV conduction may occur (Figure 6.27). As in atrial flutter, carotid sinus massage is often helpful in the diagnosis. Again like atrial flutter, atrial activity is often best seen in lead V1.

Causes

Atrial tachycardia with AV block is commonly due to digoxin toxicity (Figure 6.28). The arrhythmia is often referred to as 'paroxysmal atrial tachycardia with block', being abbreviated to PATB. The term paroxysmal is inappropriate; particularly in the context of digoxin toxicity, the arrhythmia is usually sustained.

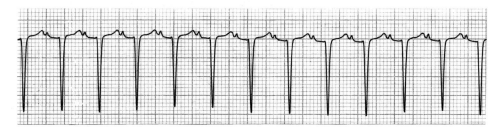

Figure 6.27 Lead V1. Atrial tachycardia with 1:1 AV conduction

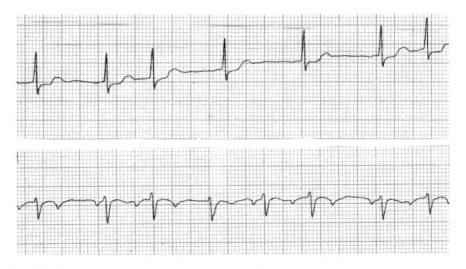

Figure 6.28 Atrial tachycardia (leads II and V1) in a patient with digoxin toxicity. Lead II suggests atrial fibrillation but V1 clearly shows atrial tachycardia with Mobitz I AV block

Other causes include cardiomyopathy, chronic ischaemic heart disease, rheumatic heart disease and sick sinus syndrome.

Treatment

If the patient is receiving digoxin, toxicity should be suspected and the drug discontinued. When the patient has not had digoxin, this drug may be used to control the ventricular rate.

If a return to sinus rhythm is required, cardioversion or rapid atrial pacing should be performed.

Main points

- There are several different tachycardias of supraventricular origin. For correct management, it is necessary to determine with which tachycardia one is dealing.
- QRS duration during tachycardia will be normal unless there is pre-existing or rate-related bundle branch block.
- AV re-entrant tachycardia requires the presence of a second connection between atria and ventricles in addition to the AV node. Usually structural heart disease is absent. The ventricular rhythm is regular. Atrial activity, if seen, will be in the form of an inverted P wave after each QRS complex.
- Atrial fibrillation, flutter and tachycardia are due to rapid atrial activity and are often associated with cardiac or extra-cardiac disease.
- Atrial fibrillation is characterized by a totally irregular ventricular rhythm. Usually AV nodal-blocking drugs are used to control the ventricular response. Though cardioversion often restores sinus rhythm, there is a high relapse rate.
- The diagnosis of atrial flutter is based on the finding of atrial activity at a rate of approximately 300/minute. Lead V1 is often the best lead for demonstrating atrial flutter: when there is 2:1 AV conduction, alternate F waves will be superimposed on ventricular T waves. Where possible, a return to sinus rhythm should be sought.
- Atrial tachycardia is similar to flutter but the atrial rate is 120 – 250/min.

Pre-excitation syndromes

In the normal heart, only the AV node can conduct atrial impulses to the ventricles. In the pre-excitation syndromes there is an additional connection between atria and ventricles. Unlike the AV node, the accessory connection does not delay conduction between atria and ventricles. Thus atrial impulses will be transmitted more quickly by the accessory connection and will initiate ventricular activation before the atrial impulse has traversed the AV node; hence the term 'pre-excitation'.

The main types of pre-excitation are the Wolff–Parkinson–White and the Lown–Ganong–Levine syndromes.

Wolff–Parkinson–White syndrome

The characteristics of the syndrome are a short PR interval, a widened QRS complex due to the presence of a delta wave, and paroxysmal tachycardia (Figure 7.1).

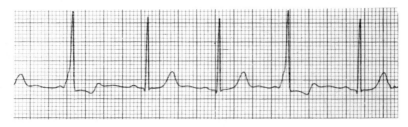

Figure 7.1 Wolff–Parkinson–White syndrome. In this patient, the accessory pathway conducts intermittently. The second, third and fifth complexes are normal whereas the first and fourth complexes show the characteristic short PR interval and delta wave. By comparing pre-excited and normal beats, it can be seen how the delta wave both shortens the PR interval and broadens the ventricular complex

The syndrome is the result of an accessory connection between atrial and ventricular myocardium. This connection, a strand of ordinary myocardium, was called a bundle of Kent but is now referred to as an accessory AV pathway.

Normally the atria become electrically isolated from the ventricles during foetal development, apart from the AV junction (i.e. AV node plus bundle of His). Incomplete separation leads to an accessory AV pathway. The pathway may be situated anywhere across the groove between atria and ventricles. The most common site is the left free wall of the heart. Other locations are postero-septal, right free wall and antero-septal. In a minority of patients there is more than one accessory pathway.

Approximately 1.5 in each thousand of the population have the electrocardiographic signs of Wolff–Parkinson–White syndrome; two-thirds of whom will experience cardiac arrhythmias. The syndrome is more common in young people. It has been suggested that with age fibrosis may develop in the atrioventricular groove and block an accessory pathway.

ECG characteristics

The accessory AV pathway is able to conduct an atrial impulse to the ventricles more quickly than the AV node. However, once the impulse reaches the ventricles further conduction is slow because the pathway connects to ordinary myocardium rather than the specialized conducting system.

During sinus rhythm, an atrial impulse will reach the ventricles via both the accessory pathway and the normal AV node. Because the latter pathway conducts more slowly, initial ventricular activation is solely due to accessory pathway conduction which results in ventricular pre-excitation and thus a shortened PR interval. Because the accessory pathway is not connected to specialized conducting tissue, early ventricular activation will be relatively slow, leading to slurring of the ventricular complex, i.e. the delta wave. Once the atrial impulse has traversed the AV node, further ventricular activation will proceed normally. During sinus rhythm, therefore, the ventricular complex is a fusion between delta wave and normal QRS complex (Figure 7.1).

The syndrome is classified into types A and B, depending on the ventricular complex in lead Vl. If predominantly positive, it is type A and if negative, type B (Figures 7.2 and 7.3).

Two main arrhythmias can occur in patients with the Wolff–Parkinson–White syndrome: atrial fibrillation and, more commonly, atrioventricular re-entrant tachycardia.

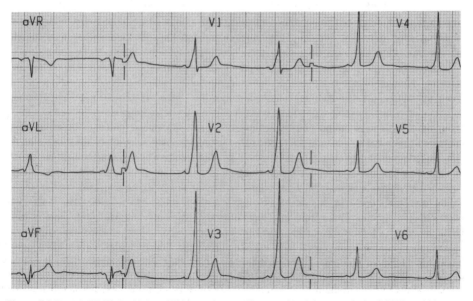

Figure 7.2 Type A Wolff–Parkinson–White syndrome. (The negative delta wave in lead AVF could be misinterpreted as a Q wave due to inferior myocardial infarction)

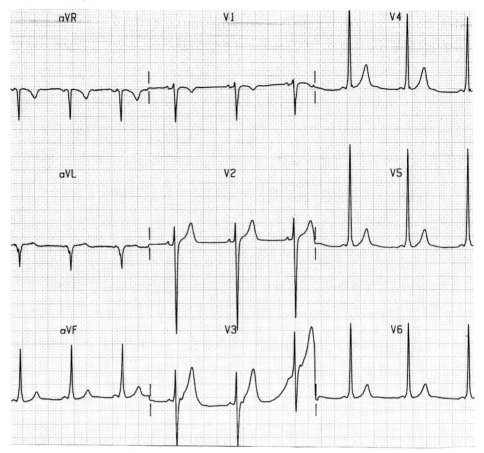

Figure 7.3 Type B Wolff–Parkinson–White syndrome

Atrial fibrillation

In patients without pre-excitation the AV node protects the ventricles from the rapid atrial activity during atrial fibrillation (350–600 impulses/min). In the Wolff–Parkinson–White syndrome the accessory pathway provides an additional route of access to the ventricles and can in some patients conduct very frequently. As a result, ventricular rates during atrial fibrillation are often very fast. Usually, most conducted impulses reach the ventricles via the accessory pathway and therefore lead to delta waves. The minority of impulses which reach the ventricles via the AV node produce normal QRS complexes. The resultant ECG will show the totally irregular ventricular response which is characteristic of atrial fibrillation. Some ventricular complexes will be normal; most will be delta waves (Figures 7.4 and 7.5).

A very rapid ventricular response to atrial fibrillation may cause heart failure or shock. If the ventricles are stimulated at a very fast rate there is a risk of ventricular fibrillation. The risk mainly affects those patients where the minimum interval between delta waves during atrial fibrillation is less than 250 ms (Figure 7.6).

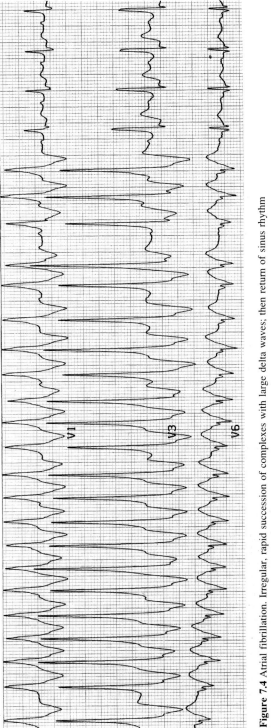

Figure 7.4 Atrial fibrillation. Irregular, rapid succession of complexes with large delta waves; then return of sinus rhythm

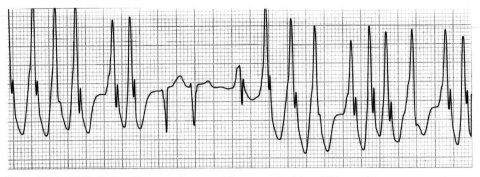

Figure 7.5 Atrial fibrillation. Most complexes are delta waves; the 7th and 8th complexes are narrow due to conduction via the AV node

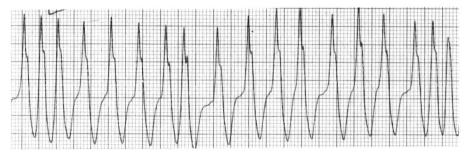

Figure 7.6 Atrial fibrillation with a very rapid ventricular response (lead V1). The minimum interval between delta waves is 180 ms. The totally irregular response excludes a diagnosis of ventricular tachycardia

Atrioventricular re-entrant tachycardia

The AV node and accessory pathway differ in the time they take to recover after excitation. Usually, the AV node recovers first. If an atrial ectopic beat arises during sinus rhythm when the AV node has recovered but the accessory pathway is not yet capable of conduction, the resultant ventricular complex will clearly not have a delta wave and will be narrow. By the time the premature atrial impulse has traversed the AV junction and stimulated the ventricles, the accessory pathway will have recovered and will be able to conduct the impulse back to the atria. When the impulse reaches the atria the AV junction will again be able to conduct and hence the impulse can repeatedly circulate between atria and ventricles, leading to an AV re-entrant tachycardia. Similarly, a ventricular ectopic beat during sinus rhythm can be conducted to the atria via the accessory pathway and thereby initiate AV re-entrant tachycardia.

The ECG during tachycardia will show narrow ventricular complexes (unless there is rate related bundle branch block) in rapid, regular succession (Figure 7.7).

Unlike atrial fibrillation, there will be no delta waves and, thus, there will be no clue from the ventricular complexes during tachycardia that the patient has Wolff–Parkinson–White syndrome. However, the timing of atrial activity during tachycardia, if identifiable, may point to the tachycardia mechanism. When the tachycardia is due to two pathways within the AV node, i.e. intra AV nodal tachycardia (see Chapter 6), an inverted P wave immediately follows or is superimposed on the QRS complex because the re-entrant circuit is small. In contrast, the re-entrant circuit is larger in the Wolff–Parkinson–White

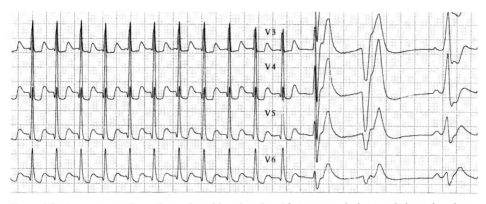

Figure 7.7 AV re-entrant tachycardia terminated by adenosine. After two ventricular ectopic beats there is a sinus beat with short PR interval and delta wave

syndrome because the accessory AV pathway is some distance from the AV junction. It therefore takes longer for an impulse to circulate and re-enter the atria. Hence the inverted P wave occurs roughly halfway between QRS complexes (Figure 7.8).

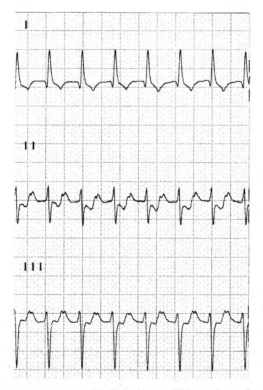

Figure 7.8 AV re-entrant tachycardia due to Wolff–Parkinson–White syndrome. Inverted P waves can be seen halfway between QRS complexes.

Concealed pre-excitation

Many patients with AV re-entrant tachycardia do not have signs of pre-excitation during sinus rhythm but have been found to have a 'concealed' accessory pathway when studied by intracardiac electrophysiological testing.

Concealed accessory pathways can transmit impulses from ventricles to atria and therefore can facilitate re-entrant tachycardia, but cannot conduct from atria to ventricles and thus there will be no delta wave or PR interval shortening during sinus rhythm.

Concealed pre-excitation should be suspected when, during tachycardia, an inverted P wave is seen halfway between QRS complexes. If inverted in lead I, the accessory pathway is likely to be left-sided (Figure 7.8).

Antidromic tachycardia

Antidromic AV re-entrant tachycardia is less common than the above-mentioned form of AV re-entrant tachycardia (termed orthodromic). The circulating impulse travels in the opposite direction so conduction from atria to ventricles is over the accessory AV pathway and return to the atria is via the AV node. Consequently, ventricular complexes will be in the form of large delta waves (Figure 7.9).

Treatment

'What is the treatment for Wolff–Parkinson–White syndrome?' is a common question. There is no specific 'best' therapy for this syndrome.

AV re-entrant tachycardia

Methods for the termination and prevention AV re-entrant tachycardia are appropriate whether or not the patient has pre-excitation during sinus rhythm (see Chapter 6).

Atrial fibrillation

During atrial fibrillation, most atrial impulses reach the ventricles via the accessory AV pathway. Thus AV nodal-blocking drugs such as digoxin and verapamil are of little use during atrial fibrillation in the Wolff–Parkinson–White syndrome. Indeed, both digoxin and verapamil can increase the frequency of conduction in the accessory pathway and therefore lead to a faster ventricular rate. These drugs should not be used in those patients who are capable of a rapid ventricular response in case a dangerously fast ventricular rate develops. In patients in whom atrial fibrillation has never occurred, and thus a fast response has not been excluded, the drugs should be avoided.

The simplest method of terminating atrial fibrillation is cardioversion, but this is not appropriate if the arrhythmia is frequently recurrent. If drugs are to be used, they must slow conduction in the accessory pathway, e.g. intravenous sotalol, flecainide, disopyramide or amiodarone. These drugs will slow the ventricular response to atrial fibrillation and will often restore sinus rhythm (Figure 7.10).

For prevention of atrial fibrillation, oral sotalol, flecainide, disopyramide or amiodarone are effective. In patients with a dangerously fast ventricular response to atrial fibrillation, the arrhythmia can be initiated by rapid atrial pacing once the patient is on anti-arrhythmic therapy to ensure the drug will slow the ventricular rate.

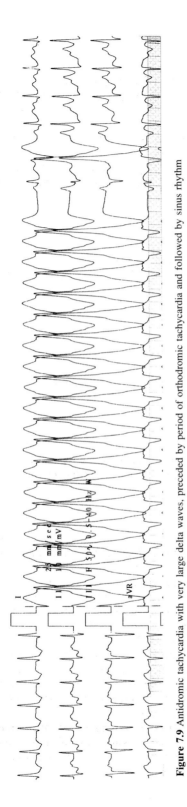

Figure 7.9 Antidromic tachycardia with very large delta waves, preceded by period of orthodromic tachycardia and followed by sinus rhythm

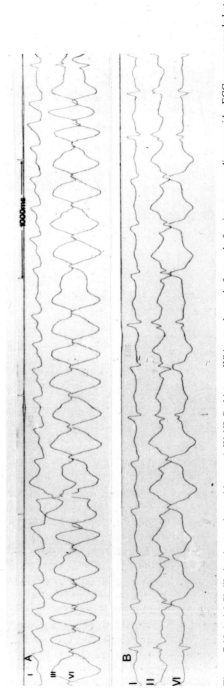
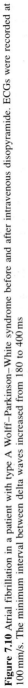

Figure 7.10 Atrial fibrillation in a patient with type A Wolff–Parkinson–White syndrome before and after intravenous disopyramide. ECGs were recorded at 100 mm/s. The minimum interval between delta waves increased from 180 to 400 ms

Ablation of the accessory pathway may be necessary when drugs are ineffective or cannot be tolerated, especially if the ventricular response is very fast.

Lown–Ganong–Levine syndrome

The characteristics of the syndrome are a short PR interval, a normal QRS complex and paroxysmal tachycardia.

In this pre-excitation syndrome there is an additional AV connection between atrial myocardium and the bundle of His, which therefore bypasses the AV node. Thus an atrial impulse will reach the ventricles without the normal delay and lead to a very short PR interval. Because the tract is connected to the bundle of His, ventricular activation will be normal and, therefore, there will not be a delta wave (Figure 7.11).

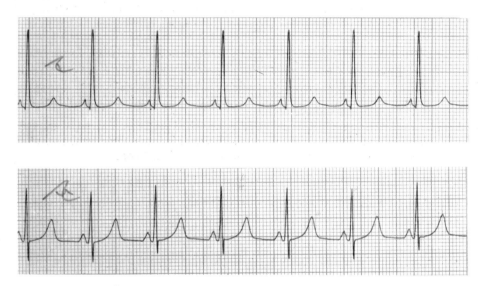

Figure 7.11 Lown–Ganong–Levine syndrome (leads I and II). The PR interval is short but the QRS complex is normal

Patients with this syndrome are prone to episodes of AV re-entrant tachycardia which should be treated in the usual way.

Not all patients with a short PR interval have an AV nodal bypass tract or are prone by paroxysmal tachycardia.

Main points

- The Wolff–Parkinson–White syndrome is characterized by a short PR interval and a widened QRS complex due to presence of a delta wave. It is caused by an accessory AV pathway (bundle of Kent), which connects atrial and ventricular myocardium, bypassing the AV junction.
- Two main arrhythmias can occur: AV re-entrant tachycardia and atrial fibrillation.
- During atrioventricular re-entrant tachycardia, there will be no delta waves and thus no evidence from the ventricular complex of pre-excitation. Treatment is the same whether or not there is pre-excitation.
- During atrial fibrillation, most ventricular complexes are broad due to the presence of large delta waves. The ventricular rate is often very fast and there is a risk of ventricular fibrillation when the minimum interval between delta waves during atrial fibrillation is less than 250 ms. If the hallmark of atrial fibrillation (i.e. a totally irregular rhythm) is ignored, the arrhythmia may be mistaken for ventricular tachycardia.
- Since most atrial impulses are conducted to the ventricles via the accessory AV pathway during atrial fibrillation, AV nodal-blocking drugs (digoxin, verapamil) are not helpful. Cardioversion is the simplest method for termination of atrial fibrillation. If a drug is used, it should slow conduction in the accessory pathway (e.g. sotalol, flecainide and amiodarone).
- The Lown–Ganong–Levine syndrome is characterized by a short PR interval, normal QRS complex and paroxysmal tachycardia. It is caused by an additional AV connection between atrial myocardium and the bundle of His.

Tachycardias with broad ventricular complexes

Causes of a broad complex tachycardia

Tachycardias of supraventricular origin sometimes have broad ventricular complexes. Thus, they may mimic ventricular tachycardia. Now that this is widely appreciated, the tendency is to misinterpret ventricular tachycardia as supraventricular, rather than the reverse.

Tachycardias with broad ventricular complexes can be due to:

1. Ventricular tachycardia.
2. Supraventricular tachycardia when bundle branch block has already been present during sinus rhythm.
3. Supraventricular tachycardia with rate-related bundle branch block, i.e. bundle branch block develops during tachycardia.
4. The Wolff–Parkinson–White syndrome when atrial impulses during atrial flutter or fibrillation are conducted to the ventricles by the accessory AV pathway or in the uncommon 'antidromic' form of AV re-entrant tachycardia when AV conduction is over the accessory pathway.

Several pointers are used to distinguish a supraventricular tachycardia with broad ventricular complexes from ventricular tachycardia:

Useless guidelines

It is often said that whereas ventricular tachycardia leads to major haemodynamic disturbance, supraventricular tachycardia does not. This is wrong. Sometimes ventricular tachycardia causes few or even no symptoms, whereas supraventricular tachycardia, if very fast or in the presence of underlying heart disease, can cause shock or heart failure.

Another widely quoted but incorrect rule is that whereas supraventricular tachycardia is regular, ventricular tachycardia is slightly irregular.

Because verapamil may terminate supraventricular tachycardia or slow the ventricular response to atrial fibrillation or flutter, it has been used as a 'therapeutic' test of the origin of tachycardia. However, dangerous hypotension may result when the drug is given during ventricular tachycardia. Never use verapamil to try to establish the origin of a broad complex tachycardia.

Useful guidelines

Clinical circumstances

Myocardial damage caused by coronary artery disease, cardiomyopathy or by other diseases may cause ventricular tachycardia. On the other hand, myocardial damage is not going to create the additional electrical connection between atria and ventricles which is necessary to facilitate an AV re-entrant tachycardia. Thus, a broad QRS tachycardia in a patient known to have myocardial damage is likely to be ventricular in origin.

Atrial flutter and tachycardia may occur in patients with myocardial damage and may lead to a regular ventricular rhythm with bundle branch block, but there are characteristic features (see Chapter 6) which should lead to their identification. Atrial fibrillation is totally irregular and should never get confused with ventricular tachycardia.

Independent atrial activity

If there is direct (Figure 8.1) or indirect (Figure 8.2) evidence of independent atrial activity then supraventricular tachycardia is excluded. As discussed in Chapter 5, scrutiny of several ECG leads may be necessary to identify evidence of atrial activity (Figure 8.3). Wherever possible, a 12-lead ECG during tachycardia should be acquired.

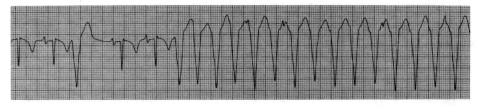

Figure 8.1 The second ventricular ectopic beat initiates ventricular tachycardia. Independent atrial activity can be seen

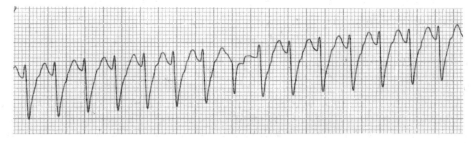

Figure 8.2 Ventricular tachycardia (lead II). The eighth complex is a capture beat

Occasionally, independent atrial activity can only be demonstrated by recording an atrial electrocardiogram simultaneously with a surface ECG (Figure 8.4). An atrial electrogram can be obtained by passing a transvenous electrode to the right atrium or by using an oesophageal electrode positioned behind the left atrium.

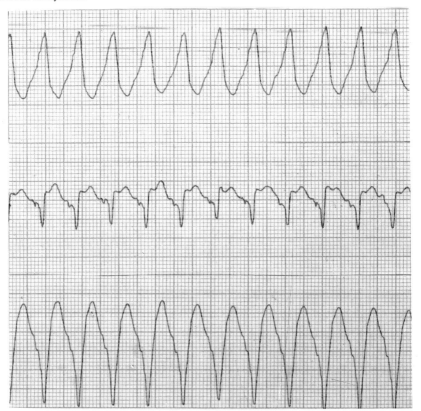

Figure 8.3 Advantage of simultaneous recording of ECG leads (I,II,III). Lead II suggests that there may be a P wave before each QRS complex and thus that the tachycardia is supraventricular in origin rather than ventricular. However, comparison with other leads indicates that the 'P' wave is in fact the initial vector of the ventricular complex

Carotid sinus massage

Carotid sinus massage can transiently slow AV node conduction and may thus terminate an AV re-entrant tachycardia. If a reduction in ventricular rate occurs during massage but sinus rhythm does not return, it is likely the patient has atrial flutter or fibrillation. During the higher degree of AV block, flutter and fibrillation waves are more easily identifiable.

Carotid sinus massage is not always effective in supraventricular tachycardia and its failure does not indicate ventricular tachycardia.

Configuration of ventricular complex

The broader the ventricular complex the more likely is a ventricular origin. In ventricular tachycardia, the duration of the ventricular complex is usually 0.14 s or greater.

Marked axis deviation, left or right, also suggests ventricular tachycardia. Another pointer towards this arrhythmia is a 'concordant' pattern in the chest leads, i.e. the complexes are either all positive or all negative.

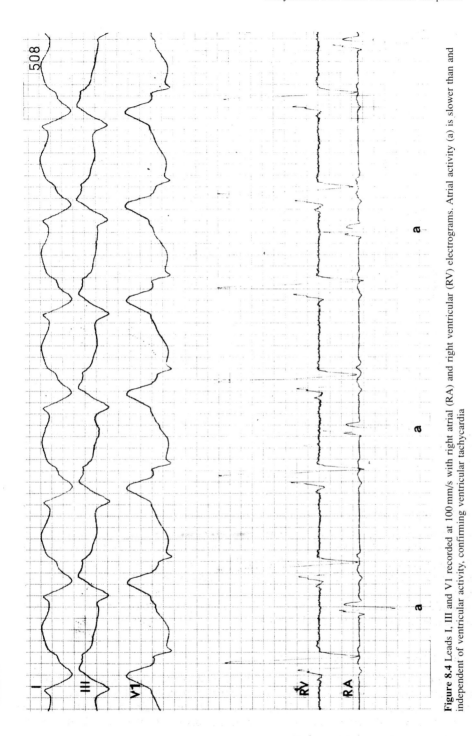

Figure 8.4 Leads I, III and V1 recorded at 100 mm/s with right atrial (RA) and right ventricular (RV) electrograms. Atrial activity (a) is slower than and independent of ventricular activity, confirming ventricular tachycardia

Retrograde concealed conduction

As discussed in Chapter 3, partial penetration of the AV node by a ventricular ectopic impulse may lead to prolongation of the PR interval during the following sinus beat. Prolongation of the PR interval in the first sinus beat after a tachycardia indicates a ventricular origin.

Ectopic beats

If the configuration of the ventricular complex during tachycardia is similar to that of an ectopic beat recorded during normal rhythm, a common origin is probable. It is relatively easy to ascertain the origin of single ectopic beats, especially if a full ECG is available (Figure 8.1).

Adenosine

Adenosine is very effective at terminating supraventricular tachycardia due to an AV re-entrant mechanism and will transiently slow the ventricular response to atrial fibrillation and flutter, making the respective atrial 'f' or 'F' waves easily identifiable. A positive response to adenosine points strongly towards a supraventricular origin to the tachycardia. Because its duration of action is very brief it is a safe drug to give (with the possible exception of patients with asthma).

However, a minority of supraventricular tachycardias will not respond to adenosine and the drug will terminate right ventricular outflow tract tachycardia. Thus response or lack of response to adenosine is a pointer towards the origin of the tachycardia but is not an absolutely reliable guide.

Main points

- Wherever possible, record a 12-lead electrocardiogram during tachycardia.
- Though bundle branch block can sometimes occur during supraventricular tachycardias, most wide complex tachycardias are ventricular in origin.
- Pointers towards ventricular tachycardia include the presence of myocardial damage, direct or indirect evidence of independent atrial activity, QRS duration greater than 0.14 s, a concordant pattern in the chest leads and marked axis deviation.
- Neither minor irregularities during tachycardia nor the haemodynamic effect of the arrhythmia are useful in ascertaining its origin.
- When supraventricular tachycardias are associated with bundle branch block the morphology of the ventricular complexes is usually that of typical left or right bundle branch block.
- Never use verapamil for a diagnostic test.

Atrioventricular block

Classification

AV block is classified as first-, second- or third-degree depending on whether conduction of atrial impulses to the ventricles is delayed, intermittently blocked or completely blocked.

First-degree AV block

Delay in conduction of the atrial impulse to the ventricles results in prolongation of the PR interval (Figures 9.1–9.3). The PR interval is measured from the onset of the P wave to the onset of the ventricular complex – whether this be a Q or an R wave – and is prolonged if it is greater than 0.21 s.

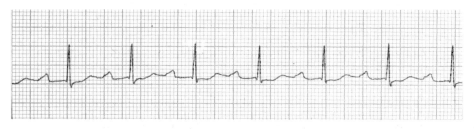

Figure 9.1 First-degree AV block (lead II). PR interval = 0.28 s

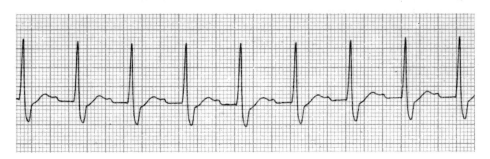

Figure 9.2 First-degree AV block and sinus tachycardia (lead I). PR interval = 0.24 s

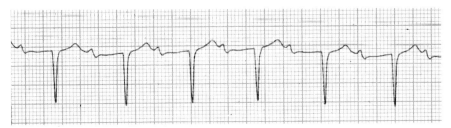

Figure 9.3 First-degree AV block (lead V1). The P wave is superimposed on the terminal portion of the preceding T wave. PR interval = 0.38 s

First-degree AV block does not cause symptoms but may sometimes progress to higher degrees of block. In young people it is usually due to high vagal tone and is benign.

Second-degree AV block

In second-degree AV block there is intermittent failure of conduction of atrial impulses to the ventricles, i.e. P waves not followed by QRS complexes. Second-degree block is sub-divided into Mobitz type I (which is also termed 'Wenkebach') and Mobitz type II block.

Mobitz type I or Wenkebach AV block

In this form of second-degree block, delay in AV conduction increases with each successive atrial impulse until an atrial impulse fails to be conducted to the ventricles. After the dropped beat, AV conduction recovers and the sequence starts again (Figures 9.4 and 9.5).

AV Wenkebach block is usually due to impaired conduction in the AV node. Like first AV block, it can be benign (particularly when observed during sleep) and is due to high vagal tone. Recent evidence suggests that Wenkebach block which cannot be attributed to high vagal tone has a similar prognosis to Mobitz II block (see Chapter 16).

The increments in AV-nodal conduction delay are usually greatest at the start of the Wenkebach sequence. This leads to the somewhat paradoxical finding that, as the sequence approaches the dropped beat, the QRS complexes become closer together.

Mobitz type II AV block

In Mobitz type II block there is intermittent failure of conduction of atrial impulses to the ventricles without antecedent progressive lengthening of the PR interval, and thus the PR interval of conducted beats is constant (Figure 9.6).

In contrast to first-degree and Wenkebach AV block, Mobitz type II block is usually due to impaired conduction in the bundle of His or bundle branches, i.e. infranodal. Thus, because there is bundle branch disease, the QRS complexes are usually broad. Block below the AV node is more likely to be associated with Stokes–Adams attacks, slow ventricular rates and sudden death.

The ratio of conducted to non-conducted atrial impulses varies. Commonly 2:1 AV conduction occurs (Figure 9.7). A similar pattern may be caused by an extreme form of Wenkebach block, so it is difficult to make prognostic inferences from 2:1 AV block (Figure 9.8). Usually, during Mobitz type II block, the atrial rate is regular. Sometimes, however, the P–P interval encompassing a ventricular complex is shorter than a P–P interval which does not. This is known as ventriculophasic sinus arrhythmia.

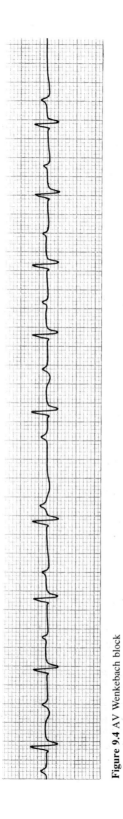

Figure 9.4 AV Wenkebach block

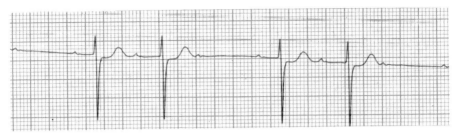

Figure 9.5 AV Wenkebach block. Unlike many textbook examples, but as often occurs in practice, the trace does not start with the shortest PR interval

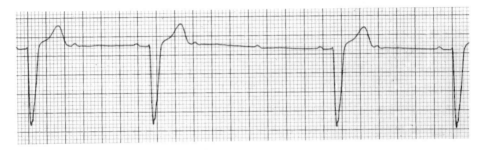

Figure 9.6 Mobitz type II AV block. In this example the ratio between conducted and non-conducted atrial impulses varies

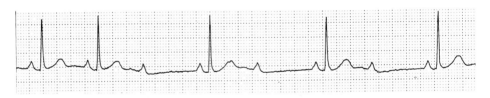

Figure 9.7 After two normally conducted beats there is Mobitz type II AV block with 2:1 AV conduction

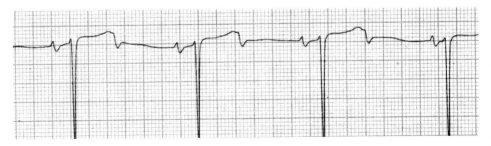

Figure 9.8 2:1 AV block with narrow QRS complexes (lead V1). The non-conducted atrial beats are superimposed on preceding T waves

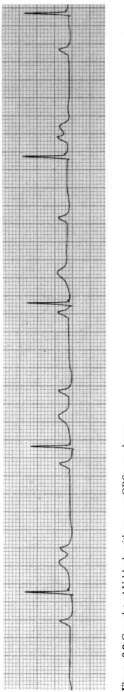
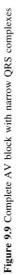

Figure 9.9 Complete AV block with narrow QRS complexes

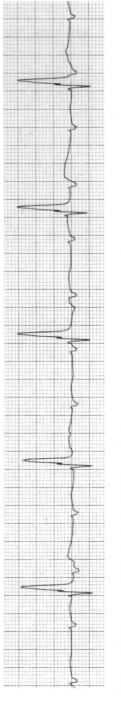
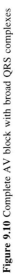

Figure 9.10 Complete AV block with broad QRS complexes

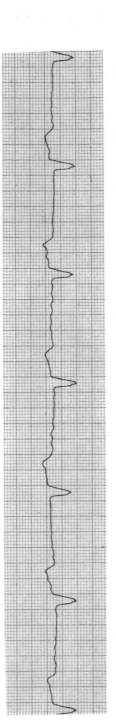

Figure 9.11 Complete AV block with atrial fibrillation

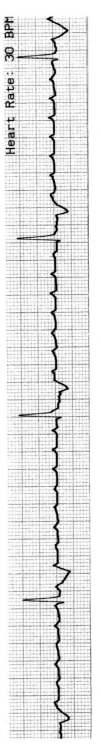

Heart Rate: 30 BPM

Figure 9.12 Complete AV block with atrial flutter

Third-degree AV block

Third-degree or complete AV block occurs when there is total interruption of transmission of atrial impulses to the ventricles. Third-degree block may be due to interrupted conduction at either AV nodal or infranodal level. When the block is within the AV node, subsidiary pacemakers arise within the bundle of His and, unless there is additional bundle branch block, will lead to narrow QRS complexes (Figure 9.9). Often, pacemakers within the bundle of His discharge reliably at a fairly rapid rate.

In contrast, in infranodal block subsidiary pacemakers usually arise in the left or right bundle branches. These pacemakers will produce broad QRS complexes and slower ventricular rates (Figures 9.10 and 9.13). They are less reliable and thus Stokes–Adams attacks are more likely.

Complete AV block can complicate atrial fibrillation and flutter (Figures 9.11 and 9.12).

Occasionally, heart block only occurs during exercise and can be the cause of exertional syncope or weakness.

Supernormal conduction

Occasionally, even during third-degree AV block, atrial impulses may be conducted to the ventricles. There is a short period immediately after recovery from excitation when AV conduction may transiently improve. This period usually coincides with inscription of the latter portion of the T wave (Figure 9.13). As a result, atrial impulses falling on this part of the T wave will be followed by a premature QRS complex.

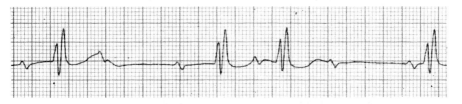

Figure 9.13 Complete AV block. There is supernormal conduction of the atrial impulse that falls on the T wave of the second ventricular complex (lead V1)

Causes of AV block

Idiopathic fibrosis of the AV junction and/or bundle branches is the most common cause. The causes of atrioventricular (AV) block are listed in Table 9.1.

AV dissociation

During third-degree AV block, atrial activity is faster than and dissociated from ventricular activity. Dissociation between atrial and ventricular activity also occurs when, often during sinus bradycardia, an escape rhythm faster than the sinus rate arises from the AV junction or ventricles (Figure 9.14). The term 'AV dissociation' should be reserved for this latter situation, in which the ventricular rate is greater than the atrial rate. If AV dissociation is not distinguished from complete AV block, inappropriate action can result. For example, AV dissociation often occurs in acute myocardial infarction and, if not recognized as such, a pacemaker may be unnecessarily inserted.

Table 9.1 Causes of AV block

Idiopathic fibrosis of conduction tissues
Myocardial infarction
Aortic valve disease
Congenital isolated lesion
Congenital heart disease, e.g. corrected transposition
Cardiac surgery
Infiltration, e.g. tumour, sarcoidosis, syphilis
Inflammation, e.g. endocarditis, ankylosing spondylitis, Reiter's
    syndrome
Rheumatic fever
Diphtheria
Dystrophia myotonica
Chagas' disease (South America)
Lyme carditis (spirochaetal infection, North America)

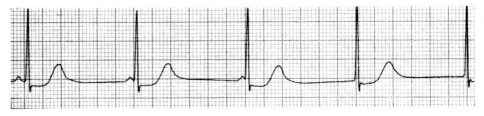

Figure 9.14 AV dissociation. Atrial and ventricular rates are 49 and 51/minute, respectively. The fourth and fifth P waves are concealed by superimposed QRS complexes

Bilateral bundle branch disease

Infranodal AV block is most often caused by disease in both left and right bundle branches.

Although the anatomical situation may be more complex, functionally the bundle of His can be considered to divide into three: the right bundle branch and the anterior and posterior fascicles of the left bundle branch (see Chapter 4).

If conduction is blocked in only two of the three fascicles (bifascicular block), the functioning fascicle will conduct atrial impulses to the ventricles and maintain sinus rhythm. Block in the third fascicle will lead to complete AV block.

Bifascicular block

The most common pattern of bifascicular block is right bundle branch plus left anterior fascicular block (Figure 9.15). The posterior fascicle of the left bundle branch is a stouter structure than the anterior fascicle and is therefore less vulnerable. As a result, right bundle branch plus left posterior fascicular block is a less common occurrence (Figure 9.16).

PR interval prolongation is usually due to impaired AV node conduction, but in the context of bifascicular block it is more likely to reflect abnormal conduction in the functioning fascicle (Figure 9.17).

Trifascicular block

Interrupted conduction in all three fascicles results in complete AV block. In many patients one of the three fascicles is capable of intermittent conduction so that, for part of the time, there will be sinus rhythm with evidence of bifascicular block.

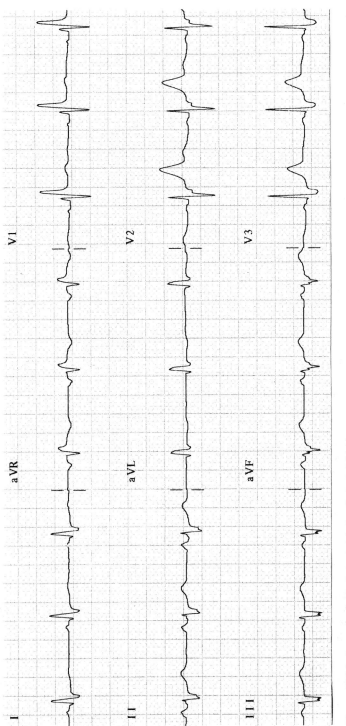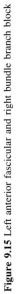

Figure 9.15 Left anterior fascicular and right bundle branch block

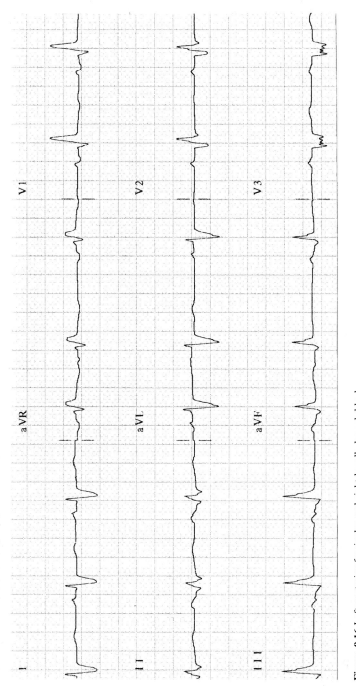

Figure 9.16 Left posterior fascicular and right bundle branch block

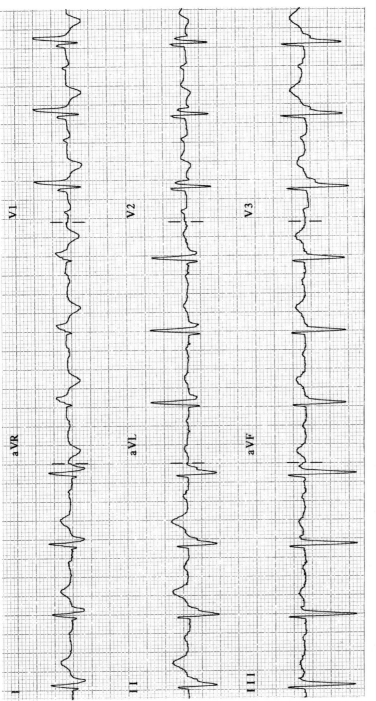

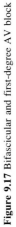

Figure 9.17 Bifascicular and first-degree AV block

The risk of bifascicular block progressing to trifascicular block is low. In patients with right bundle and left anterior fascicular block, it is a few per cent per year. The risk is increased when there is right bundle and left posterior fascicular block and when there is alternating complete right and left bundle branch block. There is little evidence to suggest that prophylactic implantation of a permanent pacemaker in asymptomatic patients with bifascicular block improves prognosis. The major determinants of prognosis are the states of the myocardium and coronary arteries.

Clinical features of AV block

First-degree and Mobitz type I second-degree AV block do not cause symptoms but may progress to higher grades of block.

In Mobitz type II and complete AV block, a low ventricular rate may cause tiredness, dyspnoea or heart failure. In some patients the ventricular pacemaker may at times discharge very slowly or actually stop, leading to syncope or, if ventricular activity does not quickly return, sudden death (Figure 9.18). Ventricular fibrillation and tachycardia arise in some patients as a consequence of the low ventricular rate and may also lead to syncope or sudden death.

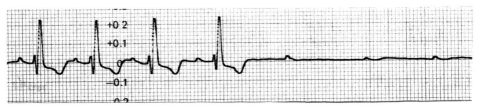

Figure 9.18 Sudden onset of complete AV block with no escape rhythm in a patient with bifascicular block

Stokes–Adams attacks

Syncope due to transient asystole or ventricular tachyarrhythmia – a Stokes–Adams attack – has characteristic features. These features are of great diagnostic importance. On the one hand, abnormalities of AV conduction (and sinus node function) may be intermittent, routine electrocardiography being normal, and on the other hand, in patients with evidence of disease of the specialized conducting tissues, syncope may sometimes be due to unrelated causes such as epilepsy.

In a Stokes–Adams attack, loss of consciousness is sudden. There is virtually no warning, though the patient will sometimes feel that he is going to faint, just before he loses consciousness. The patient collapses, lying motionless, pale and pulseless. He looks as though he is dead. Usually, within a minute or two, consciousness returns, and as cardiac action resumes there may be a vivid flush to the skin. Incontinence does occur occasionally but is not a regular feature as it is in epilepsy. Unlike epilepsy, recovery is quick and confusion and headache after the attack are unusual.

Near-syncope

In some patients the rhythm disturbance does not last long enough to cause syncope but the patient feels as though he is going to faint and then recovers. He may complain of 'dizziness' but will not experience true vertigo.

Congenital heart block

This is a relatively benign disorder. AV conduction is interrupted at the AV nodal level. Consequently, the subsidiary ventricular pacemaker is situated in the proximal part of the bundle of His (producing narrow QRS complexes) and discharges reliably at a moderately fast rate (40–80/minute) which may accelerate on exercise. Usually there are no symptoms and exercise tolerance is good.

However, syncope and sudden death do occur in a minority of patients (see Chapter 16).

Acquired heart block

Heart block complicating myocardial infarction is discussed in Chapter 11.

As discussed above, the commonest cause of heart block is idiopathic fibrosis of the AV junction or bundle branches. This mainly affects the elderly but – as with the other causes of AV block – can affect the young and middle aged as well.

The bradycardia associated with Mobitz type II and third-degree AV block may reduce cardiac output and lead to symptoms such as shortness of breath, tiredness and heart failure. Stokes–Adams attacks will sooner or later occur in about two-thirds of patients with these higher grades of AV block.

Treatment

Artificial cardiac pacing has greatly improved symptoms and prognosis. The indications are discussed in Chapters 15 and 16.

Main points

- AV block is classified as first-, second- or third-degree depending on whether conduction of atrial impulses to the ventricles is delayed, intermittently blocked or completely blocked.
- Second-degree AV block is subdivided into Mobitz I (Wenkebach) and Mobitz II types. In the former, there is progressive lengthening of the PR interval prior to non-conduction of an atrial impulse, whereas the PR interval of conducted atrial impulses is constant in Mobitz II.
- During AV dissociation (in contrast to complete AV block), the atrial rate is slower than the ventricular rate.
- First-degree block, Wenkebach block and third-degree block with narrow QRS complexes are usually due to disease within the AV node, whereas Mobitz II and complete block with broad QRS complexes are likely to be due to infranodal block.
- Bifascicular block may deteriorate intermittently or permanently to complete (trifascicular) AV block.
- Stokes–Adams attacks are characterized by abrupt loss of consciousness which lasts for a few minutes only, following which recovery is usually rapid. Patients with conduction tissue disease often experience 'near-syncope' as well as episodes of complete loss of consciousness.

Sick sinus syndrome

The sick sinus syndrome, which is also referred to as sino-atrial disease, is caused by impairment of either sinus node activity or of conduction of impulses from the sinus node to the atria. It can lead to sinus bradycardia, sino-atrial block or sinus arrest.

In some patients, atrial fibrillation, flutter or tachycardia may also occur. The term 'bradycardia-tachycardia' (often shortened to 'brady-tachy') syndrome applies to these patients.

Sick sinus syndrome is a common cause of syncope, dizzy attacks and palpitation. Though found most often in the elderly, it can occur at any age.

Causes

The cause is usually idiopathic fibrosis of the sinus node. Coronary heart disease, cardiomyopathy, myocarditis, digoxin or quinidine toxicity, or cardiac surgery, especially atrial septal defect repair, can also cause the syndrome. Sometimes, anti-arrhythmic drugs may precipitate an otherwise latent disorder.

ECG characteristics

Any of the following rhythms can occur. They are often intermittent, normal sinus rhythm being present for most of the time.

Sinus bradycardia

Sinus bradycardia is a common finding in the sick sinus syndrome. The rate may fall as low as 30 beats/minute (Figure 10.1).

Sinus arrest

Sinus arrest is due to failure of the sinus node to activate the atria. The result is absence of normal P waves (Figures 10.2 and 10.3).

Sino-atrial block

Sino-atrial block occurs when sinus node impulses fail to traverse the junction between the node and surrounding atrial myocardium. Like atrioventricular block, sino-atrial block can

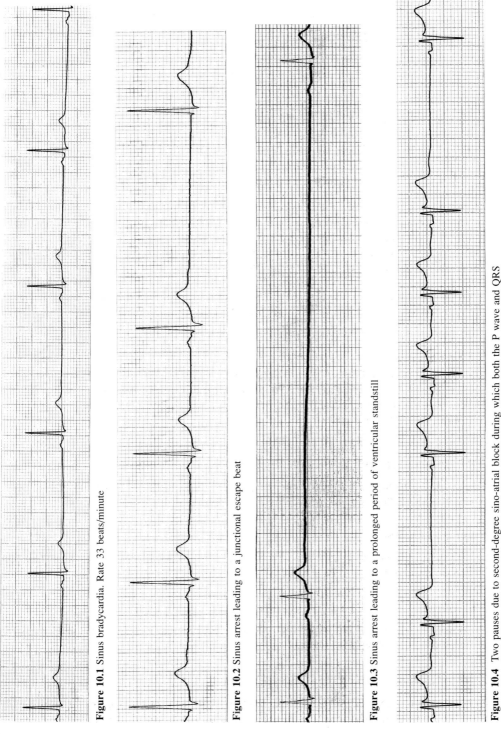

Figure 10.1 Sinus bradycardia. Rate 33 beats/minute

Figure 10.2 Sinus arrest leading to a junctional escape beat

Figure 10.3 Sinus arrest leading to a prolonged period of ventricular standstill

Figure 10.4 Two pauses due to second-degree sino-atrial block during which both the P wave and QRS complex are dropped for one cycle

be classified into first, second or third degrees. However, the ECG allows only recognition of second-degree sino-atrial block. Third-degree or complete sino-atrial block is indistinguishable from sinus arrest.

In second-degree sino-atrial block, intermittent failure of atrial activation results in intervals between P waves which are multiples of (often twice) the cycle length during sinus rhythm (Figure 10.4).

Escape beats and rhythms

When sinus bradycardia or arrest occurs, subsidiary pacemakers may give rise to an escape beat or rhythm (Figures 10.2 and 10.5). A junctional or idioventricular rhythm suggests abnormal sinus node function.

Atrial ectopic beats

These are common (Figure 10.6). Long pauses often follow because sinus node automaticity is depressed by the ectopic beat (Figure 10.7).

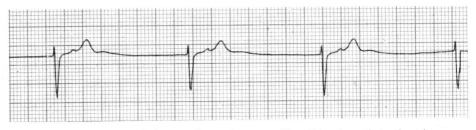

Figure 10.5 Junctional escape rhythm secondary to sinus arrest. The AV junction activates the atria retrogradely leading to a P wave superimposed on the ST segment

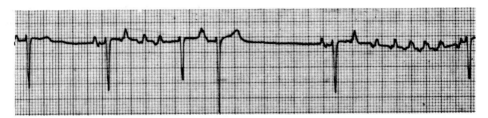

Figure 10.6 Atrial ectopic beats after the second, third and fifth QRS complexes. On two occasions brief episodes of atrial flutter are initiated

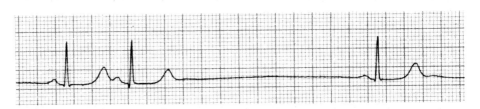

Figure 10.7 Atrial ectopic beat leads to depression of sinus node automaticity

Bradycardia-tachycardia syndrome

Several tachycardias of supraventricular origin may occur in patients with the sick sinus syndrome. Paroxysmal atrial fibrillation and flutter are the most common (Figures 10.6 and 10.8). Atrial tachycardia can also occur. However, AV re-entrant tachycardia (see Chapter 6) is not part of this syndrome.

Sinus node automaticity is often depressed by these tachycardias, so sinus bradycardia or arrest follows tachycardia. Conversely, tachycardias often arise as an escape rhythm following bradycardia. Thus tachycardia often alternates with bradycardia.

AV junction disease

AV conduction is sometimes abnormal in patients with sick sinus syndrome (Figure 10.9). In patients with sick sinus syndrome who develop atrial fibrillation there is often a slow ventricular response without AV nodal-blocking drugs suggesting coexistent impaired AV nodal function.

Clinical features

Sinus arrest without an adequate escape rhythm may cause syncope or dizzy attacks, depending on its duration. Tachycardias often produce palpitation, and resultant sinus node depression may lead to syncope or near-syncope after palpitation.

The frequency of rhythm disturbance is variable. Some patients will experience symptoms many times each day, whereas in others symptoms will only occur every few months.

Atrial tachyarrhythmias caused by the bradycardia-tachycardia syndrome may lead to systemic embolism.

Diagnosis

Suspect sick sinus syndrome when there is syncope, near-syncope or palpitation in the presence of sinus bradycardia or an escape rhythm. Prolonged sinus arrest or sino-atrial block confirms the diagnosis.

Sometimes, the standard ECG will provide diagnostic information but often ambulatory electrocardiography will be necessary.

Sinus bradycardia and short pauses due to sino-atrial block during sleep are physiological and are not evidence for the sick sinus syndrome. Furthermore, pauses in sinus node activity of up to 2.0 s due to high vagal tone may be found in fit, young people.

Ambulatory electrocardiography in a normal subject will inevitably show sinus bradycardia during sleep and sinus tachycardia during exercise. Sometimes these observations are wrongly taken as evidence of the bradycardia-tachycardia syndrome!

Treatment

Sinus bradycardia or arrest

Cardiac pacing is necessary to control symptoms. The indications for pacing are discussed in Chapter 16.

For two reasons atrial pacing, which preserves the normal sequence of cardiac chamber activation, is preferable to ventricular pacing. Ventricular pacing may result in

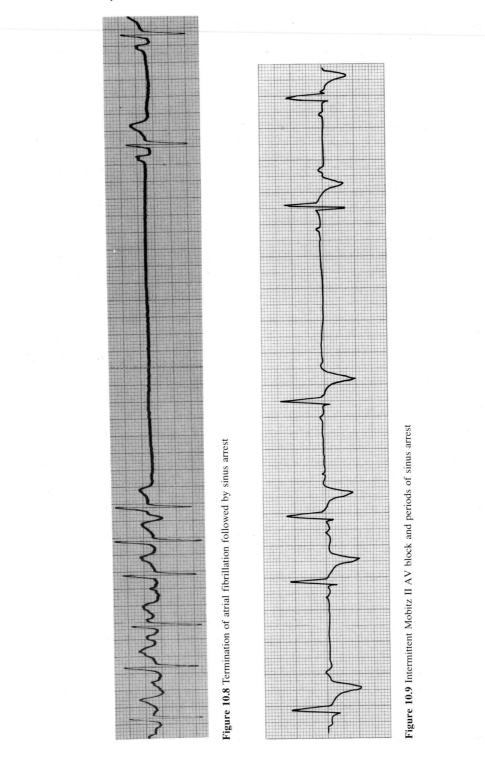

Figure 10.8 Termination of atrial fibrillation followed by sinus arrest

Figure 10.9 Intermittent Mobitz II AV block and periods of sinus arrest

hypotension and a fall in cardiac output of up to one-third (see Chapter 16). Secondly, regular atrial systole lessens the risk of systemic emboli.

The combination of sinus node and AV junction disease is an indication for A-V sequential pacing (see Chapter 16).

Bradycardia-tachycardia syndrome

Anti-arrhythmic drugs, especially beta-blockers and disopyramide, often worsen sinus node function and thus increase the risk of syncope. A pacemaker is usually necessary if anti-arrhythmic drugs are needed to control tachycardias.

Tachycardias often arise as an escape rhythm during bradycardia. Atrial pacing may prevent tachyarrhythmias by ensuring regular atrial activity.

Cardioversion may cause asystole and should be covered by a temporary pacemaker.

Systemic embolism

Because of the risk of systemic embolism, some would recommend long-term anticoagulation for patients in whom atrial tachyarrhythmias cannot be prevented. Anticoagulants are strongly indicated when there is a history of embolism.

Carotid sinus and malignant vasovagal syndromes

These two syndromes should be considered in patients with unexplained syncope without electrocardiographic evidence of sinus node or AV junctional disease.

Carotid sinus syndrome

The diagnosis of carotid sinus syndrome is made in patients who suffer from near-syncope or syncope in whom unilateral carotid sinus massage for 5 s causes sinus arrest or complete AV block for 3 s or more (Figure 10.10). In some patients, severe hypotension (vasodepression) occurs as well as bradycardia (cardio-inhibition).

Some asymptomatic subjects, particularly among the elderly, may develop a marked bradycardia on carotid massage. Carotid sinus syndrome should only be diagnosed in patients with typical spontaneous symptoms.

Cardiac pacing will prevent bradycardia. However in some patients, a vasodepressor element continues to cause some symptoms in spite of pacing.

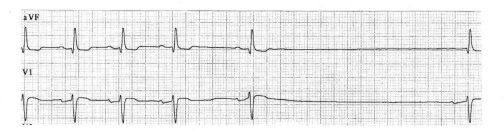

Figure 10.10 Carotid sinus syndrome. Carotid sinus massage causes 3 s sinus arrest

Malignant vasovagal syndrome

This is a neurally mediated disorder in which severe bradycardia and/or hypotension can cause syncope. It can be demonstrated by a tilt test. The patient is placed on a tilt-table in a 60-degree head-up position for up to 45 minutes. The development of severe bradycardia or asystole indicates a positive test.

Cardiac pacing should be considered but symptoms often remain troublesome due to vasodepression.

Main points

- The sick sinus syndrome is due to impaired sinus node function or sino-atrial conduction and may cause sinus bradycardia, sino-atrial block or sinus arrest.
- A long pause in sinus node activity without an adequate junctional or ventricular escape rhythm will cause near-syncope or syncope.
- The bradycardia-tachycardia syndrome is the association of both sinus node dysfunction and episodes of atrial fibrillation, flutter or tachycardia. Often, bradycardia will alternate with tachycardia. AV re-entrant tachycardia does not occur as part of this syndrome.
- Artificial pacing is required for control of symptoms due to the sick sinus syndrome and to prevent bradycardia if anti-arrhythmic drugs are to be prescribed for the bradycardia-tachycardia syndrome.

Arrhythmias in myocardial infarction

Myocardial infarction causes a wide variety of arrhythmias (Table 11.1). Some require immediate action whereas no treatment is necessary for some others. Arrhythmias are most frequent in the early hours after infarction.

Table 11.1. Incidence of arrhythmias in a series of patients within four hours of myocardial infarction

Ventricular fibrillation	16%
Ventricular tachycardia	4%
Ventricular ectopic beats	93%
Supraventricular arrhythmias	6%
Sinus or junctional bradycardia	34%
Second- or third-degree AV block	7%

Ventricular fibrillation

ECG characteristics

Ventricular fibrillation is the rapid, totally incoordinate contraction of ventricular myocardial fibres. This is reflected in the ECG by irregular, chaotic electrical activity (Figure 11.1). Ventricular fibrillation causes circulatory arrest and unconsciousness develops within 10–20 s.

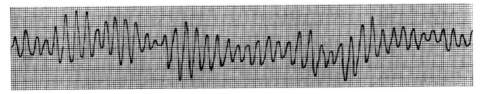

Figure 11.1 Ventricular fibrillation

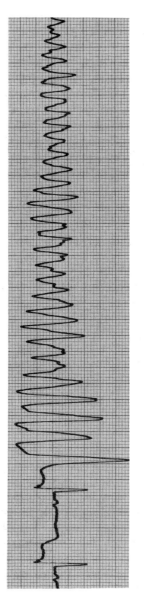
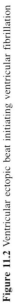

Figure 11.2 Ventricular ectopic beat initiating ventricular fibrillation

Ventricular fibrillation is most often initiated by an 'R on T' ventricular ectopic beat (Figure 11.2).

In acute infarction

Ninety per cent of deaths caused by myocardial infarction are due to ventricular fibrillation. The incidence of fibrillation is highest in the first hour after the onset of chest pain and decreases progressively thereafter. Forty per cent of deaths occur within the first hour. Thus many patients die before they can be admitted to hospital.

In those patients who reach hospital however, ventricular fibrillation and other arrhythmias are sufficiently common to necessitate continuous ECG monitoring for 24–48 h in an area where facilities for resuscitation are immediately available, i.e. a coronary care unit.

Between 3 and 10% of patients with acute myocardial infarction develop ventricular fibrillation while in a coronary care unit. The shorter the delay before admission, the greater is the incidence of ventricular fibrillation.

Other causes

Ventricular fibrillation can also occur late after infarction and, in patients with severe coronary artery disease, without myocardial infarction: it may be the first clinical manifestation of the disease.

The arrhythmia can result from other cardiac disorders such as cardiomyopathy but is discussed in this chapter because primary ventricular fibrillation due to myocardial infarction is a major cause of death in the Western world.

Primary and secondary ventricular fibrillation

If ventricular fibrillation develops in a heart that was functioning satisfactorily during normal rhythm it is termed 'primary' fibrillation, whereas if it occurs in the context of cardiac failure or cardiogenic shock, it is termed 'secondary'. Successful defibrillation is less likely in secondary ventricular fibrillation.

Treatment

Rarely ventricular fibrillation is a brief event, spontaneously reverting to normal rhythm. Otherwise, without prompt treatment, irreversible cerebral and myocardial damage will quickly ensue.

Occasionally a praecordial blow is effective. Usually defibrillation is necessary (see Chapter 14). On a coronary care unit, a defibrillator should be immediately available so little or no time need be spent on cardiopulmonary resuscitation.

A 200 J d.c. shock will successfully defibrillate 90% of cases. If unsuccessful, a second shock at the same energy level may be effective. The energy of a further shock should be increased to 360 J. The treatment of resistant ventricular fibrillation is discussed in Chapter 14.

Following restoration of normal rhythm, an infusion of lignocaine (or second-line drug if lignocaine has been found to be ineffective) is usually given to prevent further ventricular fibrillation, though there is little evidence to show that lignocaine or other anti-arrhythmic drugs are effective in this situation.

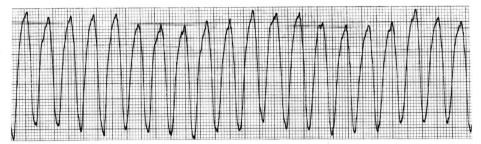

Figure 11.3 Ventricular flutter

Ventricular flutter

Ventricular flutter is a very rapid ventricular rhythm in which there are continuous changes in waveform, distinction between QRS complexes and T waves being impossible (Figure 11.3). For practical purposes, it is the same as ventricular fibrillation.

Prevention of ventricular fibrillation in acute infarction

Conventional teaching used to be that ventricular ectopic beats which were frequent, multifocal, 'R on T', or repetitive – the 'warning arrhythmias' – heralded ventricular fibrillation or tachycardia (Figures 11.4–11.7). It was common practice to suppress these ectopic beats with anti-arrhythmic agents.

However, analysis of continuous ECG recordings has shown that ventricular ectopic beats occur in almost all cases of acute infarction and warning arrhythmias are as common in patients who do not develop ventricular fibrillation as in those who do. Furthermore, warning arrhythmias may not precede ventricular fibrillation and when these do occur, staff in even the best coronary care units often fail to detect them.

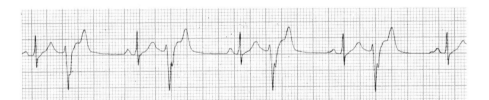

Figure 11.4 Frequent unifocal ventricular ectopic beats

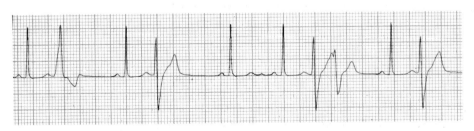

Figure 11.5 Frequent multifocal ventricular ectopic beats. The first ectopic beat arises from a different focus from that of subsequent ectopic beats. There is a couplet of ectopic beats after the fourth sinus beat

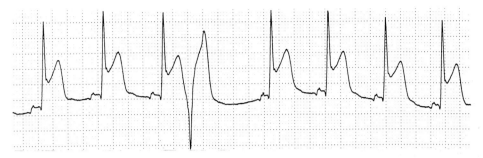

Figure 11.6 'R on T' ventricular ectopic beat

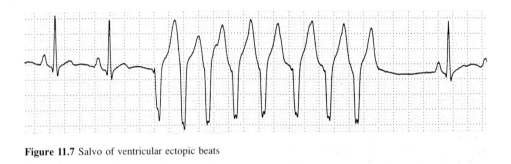

Figure 11.7 Salvo of ventricular ectopic beats

It is disappointing that, in spite of 20 years of experience in coronary care, there is no clear approach to the prevention of ventricular fibrillation. Until the situation is clarified by further studies, one of two policies can be adopted:

Prophylaxis for all patients with acute infarction

Since 'warning arrhythmias' do not in fact warn, it has been advocated that all patients should receive lignocaine. However, complex regimens of administration are necessary to achieve a consistently therapeutic plasma level of the drug. Further, with the high dosages of lignocaine that are required, side-effects due to toxicity are frequent.

Recently, high doses of lignocaine have been shown to reduce the incidence of ventricular fibrillation but only at the expense of an increased incidence of asystole.

With the possible exception of intravenous beta-blocking drugs and magnesium, there are no reports of other drugs being of prophylactic value.

No prophylaxis

Since only a minority of patients develop ventricular fibrillation, some (including the author) advocate no prophylaxis, provided that trained staff are immediately available to defibrillate if ventricular fibrillation does occur. However, there are two reservations about this approach. First, occasionally it is not possible to resuscitate a patient with primary ventricular fibrillation. Secondly, though it is widely believed that the prognosis following correction of primary ventricular fibrillation is normal, there are a few reports suggesting that it may be impaired.

Ventricular tachycardia

Ventricular tachycardia may be self-terminating (Figure 11.7) or sustained (Figure 11.8). Ventricular tachycardia may be initiated by either 'R on T' or later ventricular ectopic beats (Figure 11.9).

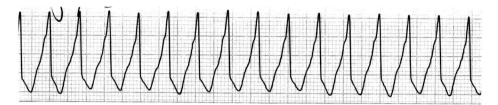

Figure 11.8 Monomorphic ventricular tachycardia

Sometimes ventricular tachycardia will result in shock or circulatory arrest. On the other hand, ventricular tachycardia may cause few or no symptoms. In myocardial infarction a regular tachycardia with broad ventricular complexes is usually ventricular in origin, even in the absence of haemodynamic deterioration (see Chapter 8).

Treatment

Only sustained ventricular tachycardia requires treatment. If cardiac arrest or shock occurs, immediate synchronized d.c. countershock (Chapter 13) is necessary. Otherwise intravenous lignocaine should be given. If lignocaine fails, second-line drugs include mexiletine, sotalol, disopyramide and amiodarone (see Chapter 12). Cardioversion may be necessary if a second-line drug fails. Overdrive ventricular pacing may help in recurrent ventricular tachycardia.

Long-term significance of ventricular arrhythmias

Early arrhythmias

Ventricular tachycardia and fibrillation within the first 24 hours of myocardial infarction are unlikely to recur after that period. Thus anti-arrhythmic therapy after discharge from the coronary care unit is unnecessary. Furthermore, most studies suggest early ventricular arrhythmias are not related to the amount of myocardial damage and are not of long-term prognostic significance (Table 11.2).

Table 11.2 Relation of ventricular tachycardia/fibrillation to infarct size and long-term treatment

	Related to infarct size	*Long-term treatment*
Early	Probably not	Not indicated
Late	Yes	Indicated

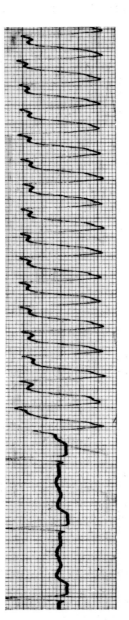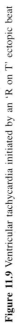

Figure 11.9 Ventricular tachycardia initiated by an 'R on T' ectopic beat

Late arrhythmias

In contrast to early arrhythmias, ventricular tachycardia or fibrillation occurring more than 24–48 hours after infarction is likely to recur days, weeks or even months later. Long-term anti-arrhythmic therapy should be prescribed.

Prognosis

The more extensive the myocardial damage the worse the prognosis. The incidence of late ventricular arrhythmias is related to the size of the infarct. However, ventricular arrhythmias are also an independent predictor of prognosis. That is, a patient with both extensive myocardial damage and late ventricular arrhythmias has a poorer prognosis than a patient with the same degree of myocardial damage but no arrhythmia (Table 11.2).

There is no evidence that suppression of ventricular ectopic beats or non-sustained ventricular tachycardia improves prognosis.

Assessment of efficacy of long-term anti-arrhythmic therapy

It is important to ensure that the treatment which is chosen is effective in preventing a recurrence of the arrhythmia. It should not be assumed that the oral preparation of a drug which when given intravenously had restored normal rhythm will be effective in preventing a recurrence of arrhythmia.

If the tachyarrhythmia has been frequent, then monitoring the electrocardiogram at the bedside or ambulatory electrocardiography are the best methods of assessing the efficacy of anti-arrhythmic therapy. Sometimes, where control has been difficult to achieve it may be necessary to accept ventricular extrasystoles and even short runs of ventricular tachycardia – provided that the rate during tachycardia is significantly slower than before treatment.

If the arrhythmia has been an infrequent event, then it is unlikely that ECG monitoring will reflect anti-arrhythmic control. Exercise ECG testing and electrophysiological testing may be helpful.

Accelerated idioventricular rhythm

This is also referred to as idioventricular tachycardia or 'slow' ventricular tachycardia. It is benign and treatment is not necessary (Figure 11.10).

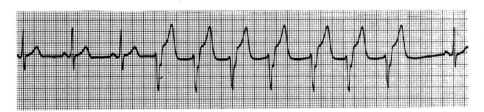

Figure 11.10 Accelerated idioventricular rhythm

Supraventricular tachycardias

AV re-entrant tachycardia can only occur if there is an additional AV connection, either bypassing or within the AV node (see Chapter 6). Thus it is very unlikely to occur for the first time during acute myocardial infarction. When supraventricular tachycardia is diagnosed in a patient with acute infarction the correct diagnosis is usually atrial flutter, atrial fibrillation or even ventricular tachycardia.

Atrial fibrillation

In atrial fibrillation, the resultant rapid ventricular rate and reduction in cardiac output from loss of atrial systole can sometimes cause severe hypotension (Figure 11.11). If shock occurs, immediate cardioversion may be necessary. Otherwise, the ventricular rate should be slowed by intravenous verapamil. If contraindicated, digoxin, a beta-blocker or amiodarone are alternatives. Spontaneous reversion to sinus rhythm is common.

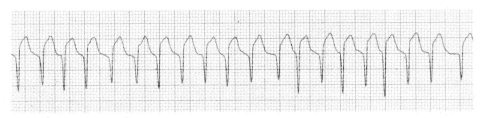

Figure 11.11 Atrial fibrillation with rapid ventricular rate in anterior infarction (lead V3)

Sustained atrial fibrillation is usually associated with extensive myocardial damage or older patients and hence a poor prognosis. Frequent atrial ectopic beats often herald atrial fibrillation.

Atrial flutter

The diagnostic features are discussed in Chapter 6. Usually 2:1 AV block occurs. Intravenous verapamil is useful, in that it will slow the ventricular rate and may occasionally effect a return to sinus rhythm. Low-energy d.c. countershock or rapid atrial pacing are often necessary for a prompt return to normal rhythm. Digoxin is best avoided because even large doses may not control the ventricular rate and will be a contra-indication to cardioversion.

Sinus and junctional bradycardias

Sinus and junctional bradycardias are common, particularly in inferior infarction (Figures 11.12 and 11.13). If uncomplicated, no treatment is required.

Bradycardia may be beneficial in acute infarction, in that myocardial oxygen consumption is related to heart rate and a low oxygen consumption might limit infarct size.

However, if bradycardia causes hypotension (systolic blood pressure less than 90 mmHg), mental confusion, oliguria, cold peripheries or ventricular arrhythmias,

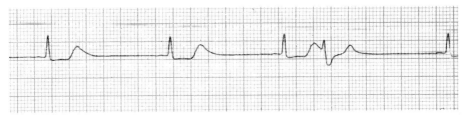

Figure 11.12 Sinus bradycardia. The fourth beat is an 'R on T' ventricular ectopic

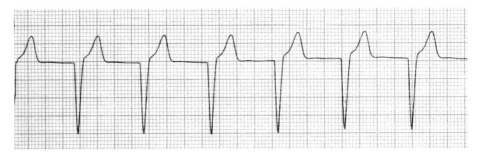

Figure 11.13 Junctional escape rhythm as a result of sinus bradycardia in anterior infarction (lead V4)

intravenous atropine (initially 0.3–0.6 mg) should be given. Temporary cardiac pacing is occasionally necessary and is preferable to frequent doses of atropine.

AV block

The management and prognosis of AV block in inferior and anterior infarction differ markedly.

Inferior infarction

In inferior infarction, AV block is common and is often due to ischaemia of the AV node. Recovery of AV node function usually occurs within a few hours or days, although sometimes it takes up to 3 weeks. Permanent AV node damage is exceptional. The prognosis for inferior infarction complicated by AV block is widely regarded as good but some studies do indicate an increased in-hospital mortality.

First-degree and Mobitz type I second-degree (Wenkebach) AV block (Figures 11.14 and 11.15) require no action other than stopping drugs that may worsen AV node function, e.g. digoxin, diltiazem and verapamil.

If complete AV block develops (Figure 11.16), subsidiary pacemakers in the bundle of His control the ventricular rate. These pacemakers usually discharge at an adequate rate. However, sometimes the ventricular rate does fall very low (less than 40/minute), when syncope, hypotension, mental confusion, oliguria or ventricular arrhythmias may result (Figure 11.17). In these circumstances temporary cardiac pacing is necessary. There is no place for steroids or catecholamines, although in the first 6 hours after infarction, atropine may be effective.

AV block will almost always resolve within 3 weeks of infarction, and it is highly unlikely that long-term pacing will be necessary.

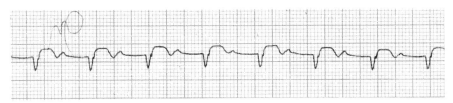

Figure 11.14 First-degree AV block (lead AVF)

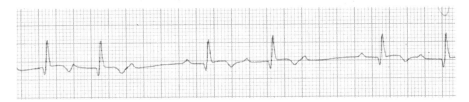

Figure 11.15 Wenkebach AV block in inferior infarction (lead AVF)

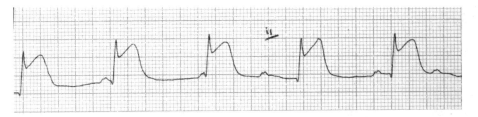

Figure 11.16 Inferior infarction complicated by complete AV block (lead II)

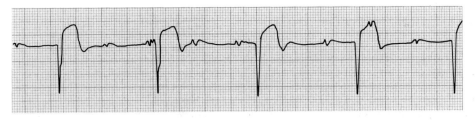

Figure 11.17 Complete heart block with ventricular rate of 38/minute

Anterior infarction

In anterior infarction, it is the bundle branches rather than the AV node which are usually the site of ischaemic damage. AV block is more serious than in inferior infarction for two reasons. First, subsidiary pacemakers which arise below the level of the block in the distal specialized conducting system tend to be slower and less reliable. Thus circulatory disturbances due to a low ventricular rate are common and ventricular standstill often occurs. Secondly, an extensive area of infarction is necessary to affect both bundle branches. Prognosis after myocardial infarction is related to the extent of infarction. Hence it is poor in patients with anterior infarction complicated by AV block.

Evidence of bilateral bundle branch damage (alternating right and left bundle branch block, or right bundle branch block with left anterior or posterior hemiblock) usually precedes the onset of second-degree (Mobitz type II) or complete AV block (Figures

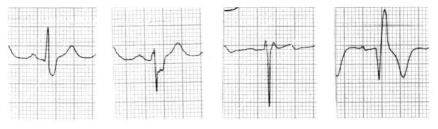

Figure 11.18 Left anterior fascicular and right bundle branch block in anterior infarction (leads I, II, III and V1)

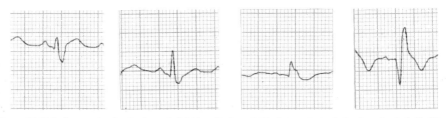

Figure 11.19 Left posterior fascicular and right bundle branch block in anterior infarction (leads I, II, III and V1)

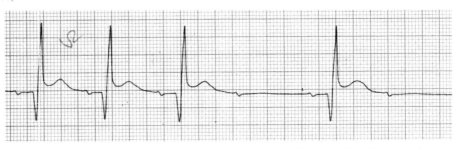

Figure 11.20 Intermittent Mobitz type II AV block in a patient with bifascicular block due to anterior infarction (lead V2)

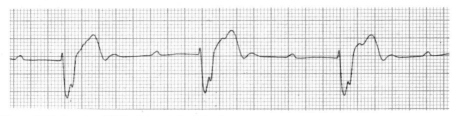

Figure 11.21 Complete AV block in anterior infarction

11.18–11.21). The chance of bilateral bundle branch damage progressing to second-degree or complete heart block is approximately 30%. The first manifestation of these higher degrees of block may be ventricular standstill (Figure 11.22). Temporary transvenous pacing should be considered if there is evidence of bilateral bundle branch damage, provided that an experienced operator is available. Otherwise the risks of temporary pacing will outweigh the advantages of pacing.

Second- and third-degree AV block due to anterior infarction are always indications for temporary pacing. Sinus rhythm often returns after a few days but in some patients AV block will persist and may necessitate long-term pacing. Mortality is high in the first 3

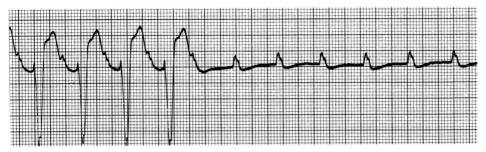

Figure 11.22 Ventricular asystole due to complete AV block in a patient with bifascicular block due to anterior infarction

weeks after anterior infarction complicated by AV block and long-term pacing should not be undertaken until the patient has survived this period.

If sinus rhythm does return, bifascicular block often persists. Complete AV block may recur in the weeks and months after acute infarction but there is no conclusive evidence to show that implantation of a pacemaker will improve prognosis. This is because the extensive myocardial damage associated with this situation will often lead to ventricular fibrillation or heart failure.

AV dissociation

In contrast to complete AV block, the atrial rate is lower than the ventricular rate and no treatment is necessary.

Main points

- Ventricular fibrillation occurs during the first hour of acute myocardial infarction in more than 30% of patients: the incidence falls progressively thereafter.
- Frequent, 'R on T' and other 'warning arrhythmias' are common in acute infarction and are not predictive of ventricular fibrillation. Anti-arrhythmic drugs are not indicated.
- Immediate defibrillation should be carried out if ventricular fibrillation occurs.
- Ventricular fibrillation or other major ventricular arrhythmia during the first 24 hours of infarction is not an indication for long-term anti-arrhythmic therapy, whereas therapy should be given if these arrhythmias occur after 24 hours.
- Atrial fibrillation and ventricular arrhythmias arising 24 hours or more after acute infarction are usually associated with extensive myocardial damage and hence an impaired prognosis.
- Sinus and junctional bradycardia and complete AV block due to inferior infarction do not require treatment unless there are symptoms, marked hypotension, other signs of shock or ventricular arrhythmias.
- AV block due to acute inferior infarction may persist for up to 3 weeks and is not an indication for permanent pacemaker implantation.
- Bilateral bundle branch damage or higher degrees of AV block in anterior infarction imply extensive myocardial damage and a poor prognosis

Anti-arrhythmic drugs

Limitations

Drugs are the mainstay of treatment for arrhythmias but their limitations should be appreciated (Table 12.1).

Anti-arrhythmic drugs are of limited effectiveness. In other words, a drug prescribed in the correct dose for an appropriate indication may fail to work.

Table 12.1 Limitations of anti-arrhythmic drugs

Limited efficacy
Unwanted effects are common
Difficulty in maintaining therapeutic drug levels
Selection of an effective drug is often based on trial and error

Unwanted effects often occur. The most common are symptoms from the gastro-intestinal and central nervous systems, hypotension, heart failure and impairment of the specialized cardiac conducting tissues. Sometimes, drugs may be 'pro-arrhythmic' in that they may worsen or cause arrhythmias.

With many drugs it may be difficult to maintain consistently therapeutic drug levels.

Considerable insight into the mode of action of anti-arrhythmic drugs has been gained, but selection for an individual patient of a drug that is both effective and well tolerated is often a process of trial and error.

Choice of treatment

Drugs are only one form of treatment and in some situations other approaches such as vagal stimulation, cardioversion, artificial pacing, percutaneous ablation or surgery may be more appropriate. A number of factors influence the choice of treatment: the type of arrhythmia, the urgency of the situation, the need for short- or long-term therapy, and the presence of impaired myocardial performance, sinus node dysfunction or abnormal AV conduction.

It is important to bear in mind whether an anti-arrhythmic drug is being given to terminate an arrhythmia, to prevent its recurrence or to slow the heart rate during the arrhythmia. In some situations drugs are given to control symptoms whereas in others the purpose may be to prevent dangerous arrhythmias.

Modes of action

The modes of action of anti-arrhythmic drugs can be classified according to their effects in the intact heart (clinical classification) or according to their effects at cellular level as established by *in vitro* studies (action potential classification). The latter classification is widely referred to, though it is of limited practical value.

Clinical classification

Drugs are divided into three groups according to their main site or sites of action in the intact heart (Table 12.2).

Table 12.2 Classification of anti-arrhythmic actions according to principal site(s) of action in intact heart

AV node
   Verapamil, diltiazem, adenosine, digoxin, beta-blockers

Ventricles
   Lignocaine, mexiletine, tocainide, phenytoin

Atria, ventricles and accessory AV pathways
   Quinidine, disopyramide, amiodarone, flecainide, procainamide, propafenone, sotalol

The first group consists of drugs whose chief action is to slow conduction in the AV node. These drugs are therefore useful in the treatment of arrhythmias of supraventricular origin but are of little or no use in the treatment of ventricular arrhythmias. In the second group, there are drugs that work mainly in ventricular arrhythmias. The third group comprises drugs that act on the atria, ventricles and, in cases of Wolff–Parkinson–White syndrome, accessory AV pathways. Thus, they may be effective in both supraventricular and ventricular arrhythmias.

Action potential classification

In this classification, drugs are divided into four main classes depending upon their electrophysiological effects at cellular level (Table 12.3).

Class I drugs impede the transport of sodium across the cell membrane during the initiation of cellular activation and thereby reduce the rate of rise of the action potential (phase 0). Many drugs fall into this group. They are subdivided into classes A, B and C according to their effect on the duration of the action potential (which is reflected in the surface electrocardiogram by the QT interval).

IA drugs increase the duration of the action potential, IB drugs shorten it and IC drugs have little effect. The anti-arrhythmic action of IB drugs is confined to the ventricles,

Table 12.3 Examples of action potential classification

I	II	III	IV

A. Quinidine
    Procainamide
    Disopyramide
    Pirmenol
	Beta-blockers
	Bretylium
		Amiodarone
		Sotalol
		Bretylium
			Verapamil
			Diltiazem

B. Lignocaine
    Mexiletine
    Tocainide
    Phenytoin
    Aprindine			

C. Flecainide
    Propafenone
    Encainide
    Lorcainide			

whereas IA and IC drugs affect both atria and ventricles. IA and particularly IC drugs slow intraventricular conduction.

Class II drugs interfere with the effects of the sympathetic nervous system on the heart. They do not affect the action potential of most myocardial cells but do reduce the slope of spontaneous depolarization (phase 4) of cells with pacemaker activity and thus the rate of pacemaker discharge.

Class III drugs prolong the duration of the action potential and hence the length of the refractory period, but do not slow phase 0.

Class IV drugs antagonize the transport of calcium across the cell membrane which follows the inward flux of sodium during cellular activation. Cells in the AV and sinus nodes are particularly susceptible. It should be noted that some calcium antagonists, e.g. nifedipine, do not have an anti-arrhythmic action.

Table 12.3 shows that the majority of drugs are in class I, some drugs have more than one class of action, and drugs within class I differ significantly in their clinical effects. Furthermore, some drugs, e.g. digoxin and adenosine, cannot be classified.

Notes on individual drugs

Lignocaine

Lignocaine is the first-line drug for ventricular arrhythmias but is ineffective in supraventricular arrhythmias. The drug is a vasoconstrictor and, unlike many drugs, rarely causes hypotension or heart failure.

A 100 mg bolus given intravenously over 2 minutes will usually be successful. If not, a further bolus (50–75 mg) should be given after 5 minutes.

Several concentrations of lignocaine are available, and disasters have occurred because the wrong concentration has been used. It should be remembered that 10 ml 1% lignocaine contains 100 mg.

Lignocaine is often used for short-term prophylaxis of ventricular arrhythmias. The therapeutic effect of lignocaine is closely related to plasma levels, which fall rapidly after a bolus injection. Thus it is necessary to give a continuous infusion immediately after the bolus. There is, however, no point in giving a continuous infusion if the bolus has failed to work or, since lignocaine cannot be administered by mouth, if long-term prophylaxis is required.

It can be difficult to maintain therapeutic levels of lignocaine. With sub-therapeutic levels, the patient is at risk from arrhythmias, while toxic levels may cause symptoms related to the central nervous system, including light-headedness, confusion, twitching, paraesthesias and epileptic fits. With conventional infusion rates (1–4 mg/minute) sub-therapeutic levels commonly occur in the first 1–2 hours after the infusion is commenced.

Lignocaine is metabolized by the liver, and where there is liver disease or where hepatic blood flow is reduced by heart failure or by shock, dosages should be halved to avoid toxicity. Hypokalaemia may impair lignocaine's efficacy.

Mexiletine

Mexiletine is similar to lignocaine in its therapeutic and haemodynamic actions but it can be given by mouth as well as parenterally. There is a narrow margin between therapeutic and toxic effects; symptoms such as nausea, vomiting, confusion, tremor, ataxia, as well as bradycardia and hypotension, are not uncommon.

Intravenously, the drug is given in a dose of 100–250 mg over 5–10 minutes, followed by 250 mg over 1 hour and a further 250 mg over 2 hours. The infusion can then be continued at 0.5–1.0 mg/minute or oral therapy started.

The oral dose is 200–300 mg 8-hourly. If the patient has not received a prior infusion, a loading dose of 400 mg can be given. Up to one-third of patients experience unwanted effects with long-term administration.

The drug is mainly metabolized by the liver and doses should be reduced if there is hepatic disease or heart failure. Approximately 10% is excreted unchanged in the urine. Renal excretion is inhibited by alkaline urine but this is not a problem in practice.

Although in the same anti-arrhythmic class as lignocaine, mexiletine may sometimes be effective when lignocaine has failed.

Tocainide

Tocainide is also similar to lignocaine. Like mexiletine it is effective both intravenously and by mouth. Its duration of action is somewhat longer than mexiletine, making twice-daily oral administration possible. Forty per cent of the drug is excreted by the kidneys and dosage should be reduced if there is renal impairment.

The intravenous dosage is 750 mg over 15 minutes. The daily oral dosage is 1200 mg. Side-effects include tremor, light-headedness, confusion and convulsions.

There have been reports of tocainide causing agranulocytosis and thrombocytopenia. In the UK it is now recommended that the drug is only used for life-threatening ventricular arrhythmias where other drugs are ineffective or are contraindicated.

Quinidine

Quinidine can be effective in both supraventricular and ventricular arrhythmias. The drug is rarely used parenterally because severe hypotension may result. Orally, its use has been limited because of its reputation for causing dangerous rhythm disturbances, especially torsade de pointes tachycardia. However, slow-release preparations (e.g. Kinidin Durules) enable therapeutic levels to be maintained with much less risk of toxicity and have the advantage that twice-daily administration (0.5–0.75 g twice daily) is sufficient.

Impaired sinus node and myocardial function are less likely to be worsened by quinidine than by disopyramide or beta-blockers. Because it has a mild anticholinergic action, AV node conduction may be enhanced with a resultant increase in ventricular rate during atrial flutter and fibrillation.

QT interval prolongation occurs with therapeutic doses, but lengthening of the QRS complex by more than 25% indicates toxicity. The drug should not be given to patients whose QT interval is already prolonged. Gastrointestinal symptoms are not infrequent. Tinnitus, deafness, thrombocytopenia and hypotension occasionally occur. Quinidine therapy can elevate digoxin levels and precipitate toxicity. The drug is metabolized by the liver and doses should be reduced if there is hepatic disease.

Disopyramide

Disopyramide is widely used for both supraventricular and ventricular arrhythmias. However, it is only moderately effective and does have significant unwanted effects.

The intravenous dose is 1.5–2.0 mg/kg up to a maximum of 150 mg, given over no less than 5 minutes. The injection should be stopped if the arrhythmia is terminated. Therapy can be continued by intravenous infusion at 20–30 mg/hour, up to a maximum of 800 mg daily, or the patient can be transferred to oral therapy. The oral dose is 300–800 mg daily in three or four divided doses. If necessary a loading dose of 300 mg can be given.

Given intravenously, the drug is more likely to cause hypotension and heart failure than lignocaine and related drugs and its use can be disastrous if the recommended minimum period of administration is ignored.

Orally, the drug's side-effects are mainly related to its anticholinergic (atropine-like) action which often causes a dry mouth, blurred vision, urinary hesitancy or retention and, by enhancing AV nodal conduction, an increase in the ventricular response to atrial flutter and fibrillation. The drug may precipitate heart failure in patients with impaired myocardial function. It may occasionally induce torsade de pointes tachycardia and should not be given to patients with QT interval prolongation. Disopyramide may worsen impaired sinus node function and is contraindicated in the sick sinus syndrome. The drug is partially excreted by the kidneys and dosage should be reduced in renal disease.

Procainamide

Procainamide has similar anti-arrhythmic properties to quinidine. It is not widely used. It has a short half-life necessitating very frequent dosage when given by mouth. Even with a slow-release preparation, 8-hourly administration is necessary. Furthermore, unwanted effects such as systemic lupus syndrome, gastrointestinal symptoms, hypotension and agranulocytosis make it unsuitable for long-term use. Impaired renal function and a slow acetylator status both reduce procainamide requirements.

N-acetyl-procainamide, a metabolite of procainamide, has been shown to have a longer duration of action and not to cause systemic lupus.

Flecainide

Flecainide is a potent drug which can be given both orally and parenterally. Its indications include ventricular arrhythmias and pre-excitation syndromes. It is very effective at suppressing ventricular ectopic beats but somewhat less so in the treatment of ventricular tachycardia.

It has a long half-life of approximately 16 hours which facilitates twice-daily oral administration. The usual dosage is 100 mg twice daily. The intravenous dose is 2 mg/kg body weight over not less than 10 minutes; it should be given more slowly in patients with impaired ventricular function. Flecainide is both metabolized by the liver and excreted by the kidney.

The drug has a narrow therapeutic range, i.e. it can be difficult to achieve a therapeutic action without unwanted effects. The most common side-effect is visual disturbance, particularly on rotating the head. Light-headedness and nausea can also occur. The drug has been shown to increase the endocardial pacing threshold.

The drug does have an important negative inotropic action and should be avoided in patients in heart failure or with extensive myocardial damage. It can be pro-arrhythmic, particularly in patients with a history of sustained ventricular tachycardia and/or poor ventricular function. In a recent study of patients with ventricular extrasystoles following myocardial infarction, flecainide was found to increase mortality.

Flecainide causes slight prolongation of the QRS complex and hence the QT interval: it does not prolong the JT component of the QT interval as does quinidine and disopyramide.

Propafenone

This drug has both IC and mild beta-blocking properties and has been shown to be effective in both supraventricular and ventricular arrhythmias.

The initial oral dosage is 150 mg tds. If necessary, dosage can be increased, after a 3-day interval, to 300 mg bd or tds.

Amiodarone

Amiodarone has several advantages over other drugs. It is highly effective in both supraventricular and ventricular rhythm disorders: even in arrhythmias refractory to other drugs there is a 70% success rate. It has a remarkably long half-life (20–100 days), so that the drug need only be given once daily or even less frequently. It does not significantly impair ventricular performance and can be given to patients in heart failure.

However, it has important unwanted effects which dictate the long-term use of amiodarone being confined to patients with arrhythmias that are dangerous or resistant to other drugs, or where the risk of side-effects is not a major consideration because the patient's prognosis is poor, e.g. the elderly and those with severe myocardial damage.

The drug has a delayed onset of action. When given by mouth, it usually takes 3–7 days before it takes effect and it may take 50 days to achieve its maximal action. If necessary, delay can be minimized by giving large doses, e.g. 1200 mg daily for 1 or 2 weeks. The dose can then be reduced to 400–600 mg daily. Once the arrhythmia is controlled, it is recommended that the dose be progressively reduced until the lowest effective dose is found. The usual maintenance dose is 200–400 mg daily. In a few patients, a dose as small as 200 mg on alternate days will suffice. With dangerous arrhythmias where a recurrence cannot be risked, it is best not to reduce the dose below 400 mg daily.

The drug is thought to be metabolized by the liver. It is not excreted by the kidneys. The main metabolite is desethylamiodarone which may itself have an anti-arrhythmic action. Very high concentrations of amiodarone and its metabolite are achieved in the lungs, heart, liver and adipose tissue.

Intravenous administration will lead to an earlier effect than oral therapy, but unlike most drugs an immediate anti-arrhythmic effect rarely occurs: an effect is usually seen within 1–24 hours. When an arrhythmia has been difficult to control, it is often worth resorting to intravenous amiodarone in spite of possible delay in action rather than to try further drugs which are less potent and which often cause unwanted effects.

The recommended intravenous dosage is 5 mg/kg body weight over 30 minutes to 1 hour, followed by 15 mg/kg over 24 hours. In an emergency, the initial infusion can be given more rapidly but its vasodilator action may cause marked hypotension. It is important to give the drug via a central venous line to avoid phlebitis. If this is not possible, frequent changes of peripheral infusion site will often be sufficient.

Short-term treatment with intravenous amiodarone is unlikely to cause side-effects, although recently two cases of hepatitis associated with the drug have been described.

Longer term oral therapy is associated with a high incidence of side-effects. The most common are corneal microdeposits and skin photosensitivity.

Corneal microdeposits occur in virtually all patients but permanent damage does not occur. The microdeposits disappear if the drug is stopped and are a useful sign of compliance. Recently, there have been a few reports of a possible association between the drug and optic neuropathy.

Skin photosensitivity to UVA radiation affects two-thirds of patients. Though only a minority experience severe photosensitivity, all patients should be warned about the possibility. If necessary, protective clothing, avoidance of prolonged sunlight and barrier creams containing zinc oxide may be recommended. Severe photosensitivity is the commonest reason for stopping the drug. A degree of photosensitivity may persist for over a year afterwards. There appears to be no relation between skin type or dosage and this unwanted effect.

After prolonged usage a minority develop marked blue-grey pigmentation of the skin, particularly the nose and forehead.

Amiodarone contains iodine and causes elevation of both serum thyroxine and reversed tri-iodothyronine and depression of serum tri-iodothyronine. These changes are compatible with the euthyroid state. However, amiodarone can cause both hypothyroidism and hyperthyroidism. If the former occurs, serum thyroxine will be low and TSH will be elevated. Sometimes there will be no clinical signs of hypothyroidism. Thyroid hormone replacement is indicated. It is not essential to stop amiodarone. If hyperthyroidism occurs, the patient will often become unwell with weight loss and other signs of thyroid overactivity. Both serum thyroxine and tri-iodothyronine will be high. Amiodarone must be stopped and in severe cases short-term steroid therapy should be given. Testicular dysfunction is another endocrine problem that may occasionally occur.

Other serious side-effects include pulmonary alveolitis, hepatitis, neuropathy and myopathy. Pulmonary alveolitis is the most common of these problems. It usually presents with dyspnoea, which may be severe, and widespread shadowing in the lung fields which can be mistaken for pulmonary oedema. Amiodarone should be stopped and short-term therapy with steroids given. Sometimes several major unwanted effects occur together. A reduction in total diffusing capacity without clinical manifestations is common.

Patients receiving long-term amiodarone should have thyroid and liver function tests and chest X-rays at annual intervals. Usually but not invariably, serious side-effects are associated with higher dosages of amiodarone.

Other unwanted effects include nausea, rash, alopecia, tremor, insomnia and nightmares which can be very vivid. The drug's class III action results in QT prolongation, often with prominent U waves. There are a few reports of the drug causing torsade de pointes tachycardia.

It is important to note that the drug potentiates oral anticoagulants: usually halving the required dosage. Amiodarone increases blood levels of digoxin, quinidine and flecainide.

With many arrhythmias, the major advantages of amiodarone, its efficacy, absence of important negative inotropic action and long duration of action, are outweighed by the formidable list of side-effects. However, most of the side-effects are reversible and the risk of them should not be a contraindication in patients with life-threatening arrhythmias, a short life expectancy or in whom other anti-arrhythmic measures have failed.

Adenosine

Adenosine is a potent blocker of AV nodal conduction. It has an extremely short duration of action (20–30 s). It is very effective in terminating supraventricular tachycardia due to an AV re-entrant mechanism and will transiently slow or interrupt the ventricular response to atrial fibrillation and flutter, making the respective 'f' or 'F' waves more easily identifiable.

A positive response to adenosine points strongly towards a supraventricular origin to the tachycardia. However, a minority of supraventricular tachycardias will not respond to adenosine, perhaps because a dose in excess of the recommended upper limit is required, and the drug will terminate right ventricular outflow tract tachycardia. Thus response or lack of response to adenosine is a useful pointer towards the origin of a tachycardia but cannot be taken as an absolutely reliable guide.

Adenosine was shown to be effective in terminating supraventricular tachycardia 60 years ago but it is only in the last few years that its value has been appreciated. Because of its very short duration of action and its safety, it is the drug of choice for the termination of AV and AV nodal re-entrant tachycardias.

Most patients will experience chest tightness, dyspnoea and flushing but the symptoms last less than 60 s. There may be complete AV block for a few seconds following termination of the tachycardia. The drug does not have a negative inotropic action. It is a safe drug to give except perhaps to patients with asthma in whom there is a possibility of bronchospasm. The drug is antagonized by aminophylline and potentiated by dypiridamole. Adenosine does cause sinus bradycardia and may briefly worsen sinus node function in patients with the sick sinus syndrome.

It should be given as a rapid (2.0 s) intravenous bolus, followed by a flush of saline. The initial dose in adults and in children is 3 mg and 0.05 mg/kg, respectively. If ineffective, further dosages of 6 mg (0.10 mg/kg) and, if necessary, 12 mg (0.25 mg/kg) can be given after 1-minute.

Verapamil

Intravenous verapamil (5–10 mg over 30–60 s) quickly and effectively slows AV nodal conduction. It will terminate paroxysmal (AV re-entrant) supraventricular tachycardia and will promptly slow the ventricular response to atrial fibrillation and flutter.

Orally, verapamil is less effective and because much of each dose is metabolized by the liver, large doses (40–120 mg tds.) are required.

Verapamil by mouth is rarely useful alone but is very useful in combination with digoxin in controlling the ventricular response to atrial fibrillation if this cannot be achieved by apparently adequate doses of digoxin alone. Serum digoxin levels are in fact elevated by moderately large doses of verapamil.

The drug is effective in two forms of ventricular tachycardia: right ventricular outflow tract tachycardia and fascicular tachycardia.

Intravenous verapamil is contraindicated if the patient has received an intravenous or oral beta-blocker. Profound bradycardia or hypotension can result and may be fatal. Sometimes, the combination of oral verapamil and a beta-blocker will cause profound sinus or junctional bradycardia. Verapamil is contraindicated in patients with impaired sinus or atrioventricular node function or digoxin toxicity unless a ventricular pacing wire is *in situ*, because of its depressant effects on the sinus and AV nodes.

Verapamil does have a significant negative inotropic effect and may cause hypotension in patients with very poor myocardial function. Two studies report that administration of intravenous calcium chloride immediately prior to parenteral verapamil prevents hypotension.

Beta-adrenoceptor antagonists

These drugs have anti-arrhythmic properties by virtue of their principal action – antagonizing the effects of catecholamines on the heart. They are most effective in arrhythmias caused by increased sympathetic nervous system activity, e.g. those caused by exertion, emotion, thyrotoxicosis, acute myocardial infarction and the hereditary QT prolongation syndromes.

Beta-blocking drugs slow AV nodal conduction and thus, like verapamil, are useful in arrhythmias of supraventricular origin. Unwanted bradycardia caused by beta-blockade can usually quickly be reversed by atropine.

Intravenous esmolol has an extremely short half-life of only 2 minutes. Its beta-adrenoceptor antagonist action and any associated unwanted effects will therefore be brief.

Sotalol

Sotalol, in addition to its beta-blocking property, prolongs the duration of the action potential and hence QT interval: it has a significant class III, or amiodarone-like, action. Unlike other beta-blockers, sotalol has a marked effect upon the recovery periods of atrial and ventricular myocardium and accessory AV pathways.

Sotalol is more effective than other beta-blockers for prevention of supraventricular arrhythmias and is also of value for ventricular arrhythmias. There are a few reports of high doses of the drug, usually in association with other drugs or hypokalaemia, causing torsade de pointes tachycardia. The oral dosage is 160–320 mg daily.

Amiloride

Recently, amiloride, a potassium conserving diuretic, has been shown to prevent ventricular tachycardia. The dosage is 5–10 mg bd. Potassium levels should be monitored. It can sometimes be effective in combination with another anti-arrhythmic drug.

Digoxin

The main use of digoxin is as an AV nodal-blocking drug in the control of the ventricular rate during atrial fibrillation. The usual dose is 0.25–0.375 mg daily. A number of factors, e.g. hypokalaemia, renal impairment, dehydration (often caused by diuretics) and therapy with quinidine, verapamil or amiodarone, predispose to digoxin toxicity and are an indication for dosage reduction.

Digoxin toxicity

Digoxin toxicity is a common problem. Over 10% of patients receiving the drug who are admitted to hospital have been found to have evidence of digoxin toxicity.

A number of symptoms suggest digoxin toxicity. These include anorexia, nausea, vomiting, diarrhoea, mental confusion, xanthopsia and visual blurring. However, none of these symptoms is specific to digoxin toxicity; in patients with severe congestive heart failure in particular, gastrointestinal symptoms are often caused by heart failure rather than digoxin.

Digoxin toxicity can cause a number of disorders of cardiac rhythm. These include atrial tachycardia with AV block (Figure 12.1), junctional tachycardia (Figure 12.2), ventricular ectopic beats (often bigeminy) (Figure 12.3), ventricular tachycardia, first-, second- and third-degree AV block, a slow ventricular response to atrial fibrillation (Figure 12.4) and sino-atrial block (Figure 12.5).

The main use of digoxin is to control the ventricular rate during atrial fibrillation. When a patient receiving digoxin for this purpose develops a regular pulse a number of possibilities should be considered. First, sinus rhythm may have returned. Secondly, an arrhythmia due to digoxin toxicity may have developed, e.g. atrial tachycardia with AV

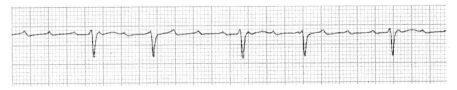

Figure 12.1 Atrial tachycardia with varying degrees of AV block

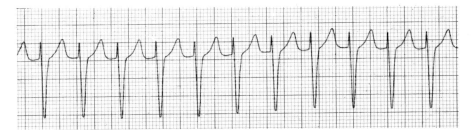

Figure 12.2 Junctional tachycardia

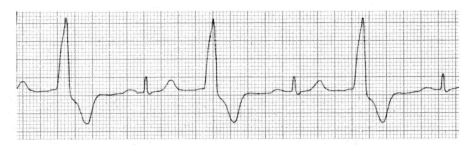

Figure 12.3 1st-degree AV block with ventricular bigeminy

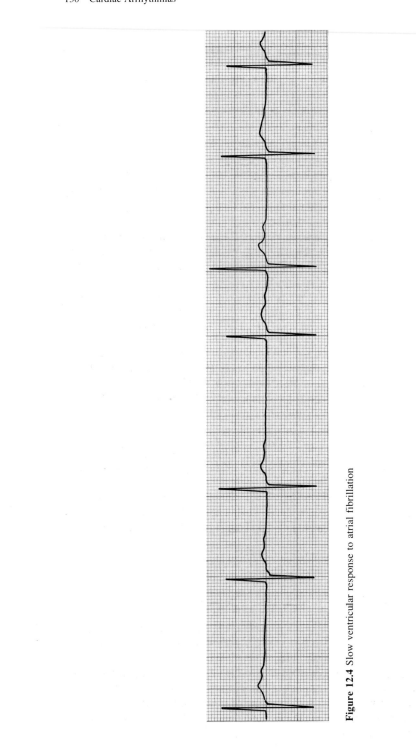

Figure 12.4 Slow ventricular response to atrial fibrillation

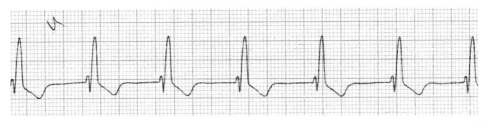

Figure 12.5 Junctional rhythm

block, junctional tachycardia or atrial fibrillation with complete AV block. Without an ECG it may be difficult to ascertain whether the regular rhythm is due to an arrhythmia or not.

Plasma digoxin levels can be measured but must be interpreted in conjunction with clinical features. Levels less than 1.5 ng/ml, in the absence of hypokalaemia, indicate that digoxin toxicity is unlikely. Levels in excess of 3.0 ng/ml indicate that toxicity is probable. With levels between 1.5 and 3.0 ng/ml, digoxin toxicity should be considered a possibility, particularly if there are symptoms or arrhythmias attributable to digoxin toxicity or if there is renal impairment, or if the patient appears to be on an inappropriately large dose of digoxin. Blood for digoxin concentration estimation must be taken at least 6 hours after the last dose.

Usually temporary discontinuation of the drug and correction of hypokalaemia, if present, are all that is required. Serious ventricular arrhythmias should be treated with intravenous anti-arrhythmic drugs. Lignocaine is suitable, although animal studies suggest that Epanutin (phenytoin) may be preferable. It has also been suggested that beta-blockers are particularly effective; these, however, may worsen AV node function and increase the risk of AV block developing.

If high degrees of AV block occur, temporary cardiac pacing may be necessary. Cardioversion is dangerous in the presence of digoxin toxicity. If cardioversion is essential, low energy levels, e.g. 5–10 J, increasing gradually as necessary, should be used and lignocaine 75–100 mg should be given.

In cases of acute overdosage, gastric lavage should be carried out. A temporary transvenous pacemaker should be inserted since there is a high likelihood of AV block developing. The heart rhythm should be monitored and arrhythmias treated accordingly.

Therapeutic range of plasma levels

The therapeutic range of plasma levels of the commonly used anti-arrhythmic drugs are given in Table 12.4. However, measurement of plasma levels is of limited use and is not often necessary in routine treatment.

If there is good evidence of a therapeutic effect with a standard dosage regimen and there are no unwanted effects, measurement of a drug's plasma level is of little importance. However, knowledge of a drug's level may be helpful with some clinical problems, e.g. when there is doubt as to whether a patient is taking his therapy or as to whether symptoms may be due to drug toxicity.

Table 12.4 Therapeutic range of plasma levels (μg/ml) for some anti-arrhythmic drugs

Amiodarone	1.0–2.5
Disopyramide	2.0–6.0
Flecainide	0.2–1.0
Lignocaine	1.4–6.0
Mexiletine	0.5–2.0
Procainamide	4.0–10.0
Quinidine	2.3–5.0
Tocainide	6.0–12.0
Verapamil	100–200

Main points

- Anti-arrhythmic drugs are of limited efficacy and often cause unwanted effects.
- Choice of anti-arrhythmic therapy should be tailored to the individual patient and depends on the arrhythmia, the degree of associated circulatory disturbance, the presence of impaired myocardial, sinus node or AV node function, the need for short- or long-term treatment and concurrent administration of other drugs.
- Drugs are usually better at terminating arrhythmias than at preventing their recurrence.
- Intravenous verapamil should not be given to a patient who has received a beta-blocker.
- Disopyramide, flecainide and beta-blockers have a marked negative inotropic action and may precipitate heart failure in patients with extensive myocardial damage.
- Adenosine is the treatment of choice for termination of AV re-entrant tachycardias.
- Intravenous verapamil will quickly control the ventricular response to atrial fibrillation and flutter.
- Lignocaine is the first-line drug for termination of ventricular tachycardia.
- Amiodarone is the most effective anti-arrhythmic agent currently available but its long-term use should be confined to the treatment of patients with arrhythmias that are dangerous or are refractory to other forms of treatment, or who have a poor prognosis.

Cardioversion

Procedure	Indications
Anaesthesia	Ventricular fibrillation
Delivery of shock	Ventricular tachycardia
Synchronization	Atrial fibrillation
Energy levels	Atrial flutter
Complications	AV re-entrant tachycardia
Digoxin toxicity	
Anticoagulation	
Implanted pacemaker	

Cardioversion is the use of a d.c. electric shock of brief duration and high energy to terminate a tachyarrhythmia. The shock, which is usually delivered by two electrodes placed on the chest, depolarizes the myocardium thus interrupting the tachycardia and allowing the sinus node to resume control of the heart rhythm.

Procedure

Facilities for monitoring the ECG and for cardiopulmonary resuscitation must be available.

The rhythm should be checked immediately before cardioversion to ensure that spontaneous reversion has not occurred.

Anaesthesia

Cardioversion is painful, causing involuntary contractions of the chest wall and upper limb girdle muscles. A conscious patient should receive a short-acting anaesthetic, or an intravenous amnesic agent, e.g. midazolam or diazepam. The patient should fast for 4 hours before elective cardioversion.

Delivery of shock

The shock is delivered by means of two electrode paddles: usually one electrode over the cardiac apex and the other to the right of the upper sternum. Alternatively, if a flat paddle is available this can be placed beneath the patient's back, behind the heart, and the second paddle positioned over the praecordium.

To achieve good electrical contact and to avoid burning the skin, electrode jelly must be applied to the areas beneath the paddles. However, it is essential to avoid spreading jelly between the two paddles. Pads impregnated with electrode gel prevent jelly being spread over inappropriate areas, including the operator!

The cardiovertor is charged to the desired energy level (see below), which takes a few seconds. The charge is usually released by pressing the button(s) on the defibrillator paddle(s). Application of the paddles with firm pressure reduces the electrical resistance of the thorax. Before discharge it is essential to ensure that no one is in contact with the patient.

If cardioversion is unsuccessful, depending on the circumstances, further shocks with higher energy levels may be tried. The heart rhythm should be monitored after cardioversion.

Synchronization

Ventricular fibrillation may be induced if a shock coincides with the ventricular T wave. For this reason, most defibrillators have a mechanism whereby discharge is triggered to occur at the time of the R or S wave. The synchronizing mechanism should be used during cardioversion for all arrhythmias with the exception of ventricular fibrillation. With ventricular fibrillation there will be no detectable R wave and thus, if the mechanism is in operation, the defibrillator will not discharge.

Before synchronized cardioversion, the operator should check that the synchronizing signal coincides with the onset of the QRS complex. Sometimes, the amplitude of the ECG has to be increased to enable synchronization.

Energy levels

In general, low energy levels are used initially. If unsuccessful, further shocks can be given at increased levels. For most arrhythmias, the initial level should be 100 J, increasing by 100 J steps to 300 J if necessary.

Atrial flutter usually responds to low-energy shocks – 50 J is an appropriate initial level. On the other hand, with ventricular fibrillation the initial energy should be 200 J.

When digoxin toxicity is likely, very low levels should be used, starting at 5–10 J.

Complications

Complications are rare. Hypotension and heart failure are occasionally produced. Enzyme levels increase in some patients, due to either skeletal or cardiac muscle damage. Transient arrhythmias sometimes occur, but these are rarely a problem unless there is digoxin toxicity.

In patients with the bradycardia-tachycardia syndrome, cardioversion may cause a major bradycardia: a temporary pacing wire should be inserted before cardioversion.

Systemic embolism may occur when cardioversion is carried out for atrial fibrillation (see below).

Nitrate patches or paste should be removed from the chest to avoid the risk of explosion.

Digoxin toxicity

Cardioversion in digoxin toxicity can produce dangerous ventricular arrhythmias. For this reason cardioversion should be used as a last resort and should be preceded by lignocaine 75–100 mg.

Because of the dangers of digoxin toxicity, it has become common practice to stop digoxin for 24–48 h before cardioversion. However, cardioversion in the presence of therapeutic levels of digoxin is safe. If the patient is receiving standard doses of digoxin, renal function and plasma electrolytes are normal and there are no symptoms or ECG findings suggestive of digoxin toxicity, then toxicity is unlikely and there is no need to postpone cardioversion.

Anticoagulation

In patients with atrial fibrillation, thrombus may develop in the atria and dislodge when sinus rhythm returns. For this reason anticoagulation should be given before elective cardioversion when the cause of the arrhythmia is associated with a significant risk of systemic embolism, i.e. history of embolism, mitral valve disease, bradycardia-tachycardia syndrome and acute thyrotoxicosis. Oral anticoagulants should be started 3 weeks before cardioversion and should be continued for 3 weeks afterwards.

Implanted pacemaker

Cardioversion may cause pacemaker damage unless the paddles are at least 15 cm from the generator and preferably are positioned so they are at right angles to the line between the pacemaker generator and the heart. Pacemaker function should be checked after the procedure.

Indications

Ventricular fibrillation

Rarely, a praecordial blow will effect a return to sinus rhythm; otherwise, immediate cardioversion is indicated. The initial energy level should be 200 J. If unsuccessful, a further 200 J shock should be given. If ventricular fibrillation persists, a 360 J shock should be delivered.

Ventricular tachycardia

Cardioversion is indicated if the arrhythmia causes shock or cardiac arrest, or if drug therapy has failed.

Atrial fibrillation

Cardioversion usually effects a return to sinus rhythm. 300 J may be required. However, atrial fibrillation returns in a high proportion of patients within a few months and often within hours of cardioversion. A long-term successful result is more likely when cardiomegaly, left atrial enlargement and a long history of the arrhythmia are absent. Treatment with quinidine, disopyramide or amiodarone has been shown to increase modestly the chances of maintaining sinus rhythm.

Atrial flutter

This arrhythmia, which is often difficult to treat with drugs, responds to low-energy shocks.

AV re-entrant tachycardia

Cardioversion is indicated on the few occasions when other measures, such as vagal stimulation or intravenous adenosine or verapamil, have failed.

Main points

- The usual positions for the defibrillator paddles are the cardiac apex and to the right of the upper sternum. Firm paddle pressure should be applied when the d.c. shock is delivered.
- Except for ventricular fibrillation, delivery of the shock should be synchronized to the R or S wave of the electrocardiogram.
- Initial energy levels depend on the clinical circumstances: 50 J for atrial flutter, 200 J for ventricular fibrillation, 100 J for most other arrhythmias.
- Digoxin toxicity is a contraindication to cardioversion. Temporary transvenous pacing should precede cardioversion if the bradycardia-tachycardia syndrome is suspected.
- In patients with atrial fibrillation or flutter due to conditions associated with a significant risk from systemic embolism, oral anticoagulation for 3 weeks should precede cardioversion.
- Damage to an implanted pacemaker can be prevented if the paddles are placed at least 15 cm from the generator and preferably positioned so they are at right angles to the pacing system.

Cardiopulmonary resuscitation

Cardiac arrest is the cessation of an effective cardiac output as the result of a sudden circulatory or respiratory catastrophe.

Patients dying of terminal and irreversible diseases will not benefit from and should not undergo the indignity of cardiopulmonary resuscitation.

Common causes of cardiac arrest

1. Acute myocardial infarction.
2. Severe coronary artery disease.
3. Myocardial damage resulting from past infarction, cardiomyopathy or myocarditis.
4. Anoxia, e.g. due to drowning, smoke inhalation, airways obstruction, or respiratory depression.
5. Electrocution.
6. Iatrogenic, e.g. hypokalaemia, or overdose of opiate or catecholamine.
7. Anaphylactic response to a drug or other allergen.

Diagnosis

Diagnosis of cardiac arrest is based on three signs:

1. Unconsciousness.
2. Apnoea.
3. Absent carotid or femoral artery pulsation.

Cardiopulmonary resuscitation

Management of cardiac arrest consists of three stages:

1. Basic life support.
2. Restoration of spontaneous heart action.
3. After-care.

Speed and efficiency in both the diagnosis and management of cardiac arrest are essential. The shorter the delays in starting basic life support and in restoring normal heart action, the more likely is a successful outcome.

Basic life support

This term refers to the combination of external chest compression and expired air respiration. Equipment and drugs are not required.

External chest compression

The heel of one hand is placed over the sternum at the junction of its upper two-thirds and lower one-third and is covered by the other hand. Keeping the arms straight, and with the shoulders directly aligned above the hands, the sternum should be depressed 4–5 cm at a rate of 80 beats/minute. Each compression should be sustained so that the time spent in compression is equal to that of relaxation.

If there is only one rescuer, after each 15 compressions there should be a pause to deliver two expired air inflations. If there are two rescuers, after each five compressions there should be a pause for one expired air inflation.

Mechanism

Chest compression was thought to work by squeezing the ventricles between the sternum and vertebrae thereby expelling blood into the arteries. Hence the older term 'cardiac massage'. However, it is now known that chest compression increases intrathoracic pressure and thereby propels blood into the systemic arteries. Valves at the superior thoracic inlet prevent regurgitation into the venous system and, between chest compressions, the aortic valve remains competent, thus preventing blood flowing back into the heart.

One piece of evidence that supports that the heart is a passive conduit during chest compression may be of practical value: rapid, vigorous coughing at the onset of ventricular fibrillation may generate sufficient cardiac output to maintain consciousness.

Expired air respiration

With the palm of one hand, tilt the patient's head backwards so that the neck is fully extended. With the fingers of the other hand, lift the lower jaw forward so that it protrudes beyond the upper teeth. Without these manoeuvres the tongue will obstruct the airway and artificial ventilation will be impossible.

Mouth-to-mouth respiration should then be given by taking a deep breath and, after pinching the patient's nose and sealing the lips around those of the patient, blowing forcefully into the patient's mouth. The patient's chest should be seen to rise, otherwise ventilation is inadequate. If chest expansion is not achieved, the pharynx should be examined to ensure that it is not obstructed by vomit or foreign material.

With one operator, two ventilations should be given after each 15 chest compressions. With two operators, each five compressions should be followed by one ventilation.

Endotracheal intubation should not be carried out unless first attempts at restoring normal heart action (see below) are unsuccessful.

Restoration of normal heart action

Treatment depends on the heart rhythm. The paddles of a modern defibrillator also function as electrodes, enabling the heart rhythm to be quickly ascertained.

The ECG may reveal ventricular fibrillation, ventricular tachycardia, asystole or, rarely, sinus rhythm. The latter may occur as a result of electromechanical dissociation, pulmonary embolism, cardiac tamponade or tension pneumothorax.

Ventricular fibrillation

Occasionally, a single blow to the praecordium with the side of a clenched fist will, if given shortly after the onset of ventricular fibrillation (or tachycardia), restore sinus rhythm.

Otherwise, the patient should be immediately defibrillated. Time should not be wasted with basic life support procedures if a defibrillator is to hand. To avoid one common cause of delay, it is essential to ensure familiarity with the controls of the available defibrillator(s).

The defibrillator should be charged to 200 J. One paddle should be firmly applied to the right of the upper sternum and the other to the cardiac apex after having placed electrode jelly or pads impregnated with electrode gel beneath the paddles. Everyone should be instructed to avoid contact with the patient who is then defibrillated by depressing the button(s) on the defibrillator paddle(s).

If ventricular fibrillation persists, a further 200 J shock should be given.

The majority of episodes of ventricular fibrillation will be terminated by the first or second 200 J shock. If the second attempt at defibrillation is unsuccessful a shock of 360 J should be given. Further action for persistent ventricular fibrillation is detailed in the summary below (i.e. step 4 and onwards).

Summary of sequence of actions from onset of ventricular fibrillation:

1. 200 J shock.
2. 200 J shock.
3. 360 J shock.

4. Endotracheal intubation.
5. Insertion of venous cannula.

6. Adrenaline 1 mg (i.e. 10 ml 1:10 000 soln).
7. Chest compression and ventilation – 10 sequences.
8. 360 J shock.
9. 360 J shock.
10. 360 J shock.

11. Repeat steps 6–10, three times.
12. Consider bretylium 500 mg (may take 20 minutes to work).
13. Change paddle positions, e.g. axilla to axilla.

The purpose of adrenaline is to increase peripheral resistance and thereby divert blood flow to the myocardium. Experiments in animals suggest that this facilitates defibrillation, though recent observations in man suggest that adrenaline may possibly have a deleterious effect. Sodium bicarbonate used to be given in large doses at the start of cardiopulmonary resuscitation to reverse acidosis but it is now appreciated that this practice is not necessary and may be harmful.

Ventricular tachycardia

If ventricular tachycardia causes cardiac arrest it is preferable to set the synchronizing mechanism so that the shock falls on the R wave rather than the T wave to avoid the risk of inducing ventricular fibrillation. Remember, if the synchronization button is depressed it will not be possible to deliver a shock during ventricular fibrillation since no R waves will be detected.

Asystole

Resuscitation from asystole is often successful when the cause is anoxia or disease confined to the specialized conducting tissues. In the former case, ventilation may be all that is required. In the latter case, the mechanical stimulation of repeated praecordial blows or cardiac massage may initiate ventricular activation. On the other hand, when asystole is due to extensive myocardial damage successful resuscitation is unlikely.

Occasionally, an ECG trace during an arrest may be flat suggesting asystole, and yet the arrest is due to ventricular fibrillation: the gain on the ECG may be too low, there may be a fault in the leads or the fibrillatory waves may be of very low amplitude. If there is any doubt, ventricular fibrillation should be assumed and steps 1–3 in the above series of defibrillator discharges given.

If ventricular fibrillation has been excluded, 10 ml 1:10 000 adrenaline should be given. Ten sequences of chest compression and ventilation should then be applied. If asystole persists, adrenaline and the chest compression sequence should be repeated three times.

If the patient is still asystolic, atropine 3 mg and then adrenaline 5 mg may be tried.

Occasionally ventricular standstill may occur during atrial fibrillation and be confused with fine ventricular fibrillation.

Pacing is rarely effective unless asystole is due to disease of the specialized conducting tissues.

Sinus rhythm

In patients with myocardial damage, dissociation between electrical and mechanical activity can sometimes be reversed with intravenous adrenaline or 10 ml 10% calcium chloride.

If cardiac arrest is thought to be due to cardiac tamponade, immediate aspiration of the pericardium or thoracotomy is indicated. Where pulmonary embolism is suspected, 15 000 units of heparin should be given intravenously. If facilities are to hand, emergency pulmonary embolectomy may be possible. Transfusion should be given if arrest is due to severe hypovolaemia.

Administration of drugs

Drugs should be given via a large vein. If necessary, a line should be inserted into a central vein. The femoral vein is a good approach, since it is remote from the area of resuscitation. The external jugular vein is often distended during cardiac arrest, allowing easy cannulation. In some patients it may be necessary to cannulate the internal jugular or subclavian vein.

If it is impossible to insert a venous line, adrenaline and lignocaine can be given via the intrapulmonary route. They should be diluted in 10 ml saline and be given through a fine catheter, introduced via the endotracheal tube, deep into the lungs. Doses should be double those used intravenously.

After-care

The patient should be transferred to an intensive or coronary care unit. The heart rhythm should be monitored during transfer. If the patient has not fully regained consciousness, the need for artificial ventilation should be considered.

Blood should be sent to check blood electrolytes and arterial gases. A chest X-ray should be performed.

Severe acidosis should be reversed with 50 ml 8.4% sodium bicarbonate.

Out-of-hospital sudden cardiac death

Sudden death due to cardiac disease is common. The annual incidence in the UK has been estimated to be 50 000. The mechanism is usually ventricular tachycardia of fibrillation. Ventricular fibrillation often results from degeneration from ventricular tachycardia rather than being the primary arrhythmia.

Coronary heart disease is by far the most common cause. Though acute myocardial infarction commonly leads to ventricular fibrillation, it accounts for less than one-third of patients presenting with sudden death. The majority have been found to have extensive coronary disease and poor left ventricular but not acute infarction. Other causes include dilated and hypertrophic cardiomyopathies, myocarditis, Wolff–Parkinson–White syndrome and hereditary prolongation of the QT interval.

Several centres, mainly in North America, have shown that facilities for out-of hospital cardiopulmonary resuscitation do save lives. As a result, information on the syndrome of 'aborted sudden cardiac death' is increasing. It is now clear that patients who are resuscitated and who have not sustained acute infarction remain at risk. There is a recurrence rate of up to 60% within 2 years.

Patients resuscitated from cardiac arrest not caused by acute infarction must be investigated to assess the need for myocardial revascularization, anti-arrhythmic drug therapy or implantation of an automatic defibrillator before discharge from hospital.

The role of drugs is usually assessed by electrophysiological testing. It is usually possible to induce ventricular tachycardia in patients with 'aborted sudden cardiac death' by stimulating the heart with precisely timed premature ventricular stimuli. Drug therapy which then prevents re-induction of the arrhythmia or at least increases the cycle length during tachycardia by over 100 ms has been shown to have a very favourable effect on prognosis. Serial testing may be required to identify an effective drug. Sometimes all anti-arrhythmic drugs will be found to be ineffective. The implantable defibrillator has the advantage of being very effective in limiting mortality but currently available devices have disadvantages as outlined in Chapter 5.

Main points

- Loss of consciousness, apnoea and absence of carotid or femoral artery pulsation are the only signs required for the diagnosis of cardiac arrest.
- Chest compression is often poorly performed. Precise positioning of the hands, at the junction of the upper two-thirds and lower-third of the sternum, is essential. The operator's arms should be kept straight by 'locking the elbows', with the shoulders positioned directly above the hands. The chest should be compressed at a rate of 80 beats/minute; the duration of each compression should be sustained and equal to the relaxation phase.
- Maintenance of a clear airway by full extension of the neck is essential for effective mouth-to-mouth resuscitation.
- If there is ventricular fibrillation, the sooner defibrillation is carried out the more likely a successful outcome. Initially, 200 J should be delivered, the two paddles being positioned at the cardiac apex and to the right of the upper sternum. To avoid one common cause of delay, there should be familiarity with the controls of the defibrillator(s) that one is likely to use.
- Out-of-hospital sudden cardiac death is usually due to ventricular tachycardia or fibrillation resulting from coronary heart disease. Frequently, there will be no evidence of acute myocardial infarction: without treatment, recurrence is likely.

Temporary cardiac pacing

The transvenous route is usually used for temporary pacing but, in emergencies, transcutaneous and oesophageal approaches are possible short-term alternatives.

Temporary transvenous pacing is essentially a simple procedure. However, complications are common because it is often carried out by inexperienced, unsupervised operators. The need for temporary pacing should be carefully considered before proceeding.

Indications

Chronic conduction tissue disease

Temporary pacing may be necessary as a first measure in patients with recent syncope caused by chronic disease of the sinus node or AV junction who are to be referred for long-term pacing.

Myocardial infarction

Indications for temporary pacing in acute myocardial infarction are:

1. Second- and third-degree AV block due to acute anterior myocardial infarction.
2. Second- and third-degree AV block caused by acute inferior infarction when complicated by hypotension, ventricular tachyarrhythmia or a ventricular rate less than 40 beats/minute.
3. Symptomatic sinus arrest or junctional bradycardia due to acute myocardial infarction.

General anaesthesia

Patients with second- or third-degree AV block should be paced during the operative period and should subsequently be considered for long-term pacing.

In the absence of a history of syncope or near-syncope, the risk of AV block developing during anaesthesia in a patient with bifascicular block is very low and pacing is not essential.

Tachycardias

Pacing is useful in terminating AV re-entrant tachycardia, atrial flutter and ventricular tachycardia. In the bradycardia-tachycardia syndrome temporary pacing should be used to cover cardioversion if required for the termination of supraventricular arrhythmias.

Methods

Temporary transvenous pacing

Temporary ventricular pacing is carried out by introducing a transvenous pacing electrode under local anaesthesia into a systemic vein and advancing it, with the aid of X-ray screening, to the right ventricle. The electrode is connected to an external battery-powered pulse generator. During insertion, the heart rhythm must be monitored and equipment for resuscitation should be available.

Subclavian vein puncture

Puncture of the subclavian vein provides the most suitable route of access to the venous system. The vein runs behind the medial third of the clavicle and can be punctured using either supraventricular or infraclavicular approaches. Only the latter will be described.

The patient should lay flat or, if possible, in a slight head-down position. A needle is introduced, through a 5 mm skin incision just below the inferior border of the clavicle and slightly medial to the mid-clavicular point, and is directed towards the sternoclavicular joint so that it passes immediately behind the posterior surface of the clavicle. When first advancing the needle it is advisable to locate the clavicle with the needle tip to avoid going in too deeply, with consequent risk of pneumothorax or subclavian artery puncture.

As the needle punctures the vein, venous blood will be easily aspirated. If there is only a trickle of blood the needle tip is unlikely to be in the subclavian vein.

Cannulation of the vein is best achieved by introducing a guide wire through the needle into the vein. A guide wire with a flexible J-shaped tip is much easier to advance around the junction between the subclavian vein and superior vena cava. The needle is then withdrawn and a sheath within which there is a vessel dilator is passed over the wire into the vein. The guide wire and dilator are then removed, and the pacing lead is passed through the sheath.

The main advantages of subclavian vein puncture are that it is quick and infection and electrode displacement are unusual. Possible complications, which are rare in experienced hands, are pneumothorax, haemothorax, subclavian artery puncture and air embolism.

Antecubital vein cut-down

It is important to select a medially situated vein. It is unusual to be able to negotiate an electrode into the superior vena cava from a lateral vein.

The disadvantages of this approach are poor electrode stability, and infection and phlebitis are common.

Femoral vein puncture

This method is very easy and quick, provided that pulsation of the laterally adjacent femoral artery is easily palpable. However, it should be reserved for short-term emergency purposes because electrode stability is poor and there is a risk of venous thrombosis. Pressure on the abdomen causes distension of the femoral vein and makes venepuncture easier.

Positioning of the electrode

If there is resistance to the introduction of the electrode into the vein, the lumen has probably not been entered. Once in the venous system, it should be possible to advance

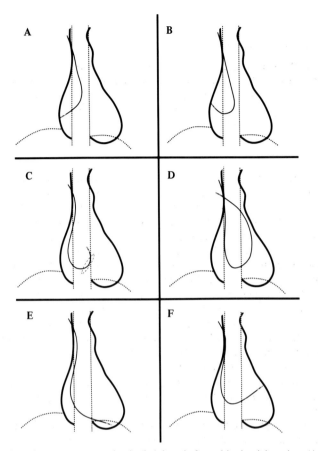

Figure 15.1 Insertion of a transvenous pacing lead. A loop is formed in the right atrium (A and B). The loop is positioned near the tricuspid valve, indicated by the oval of dashes (C). Entry into the right ventricle can be confirmed by passing the wire into the pulmonary artery (D). The pacing lead is then positioned in the apex of the right ventricle (E). (F) The characteristic appearance of a pacing lead in the coronary sinus

the electrode without resistance. If an obstruction is encountered, the electrode should be withdrawn slightly, rotated and then advanced again. Nothing will be achieved by forcing the electrode.

Once the electrode has reached the right atrium, a loop should be formed by impinging the electrode tip on the atrial wall (Figure 15.1A) and then advancing the electrode a little further (Figure 15.lB). By twisting the electrode, the loop can be rotated so that the electrode tip lies near the tricuspid valve (Figure 15.1C). Slight withdrawal of the electrode will allow the tip to 'flick' through the valve into the right ventricle.

Ventricular ectopic beats are usually provoked as the valve is crossed. If these do not occur, the coronary sinus rather than the right ventricle may have been entered. An electrode lying in the coronary sinus assumes a characteristic shape (Figure 15.lF). (A lateral view will show that the electrode is pointing posteriorly whereas an electrode in the right ventricular apex points anteriorly.) It can be confirmed that the right ventricle has been entered by advancing the electrode into the pulmonary artery (Figure 15.lD).

Once in the right ventricle, the electrode tip is positioned in or near the apex of the ventricle by a process of advancement, withdrawal and rotation (Figure 15.1E).

Difficulty with electrode manipulation can be due to poor technique. Another cause is that reusable pacing electrodes lose their stiffness after repeated use and should not be employed more than six times. If positioning proves difficult, it is well worth trying a new electrode.

Pacing

When a stable electrode position in or near the right ventricular apex has been achieved, the distal and proximal poles of the electrode should be connected to the pacemaker cathode ($-$) and anode ($+$), respectively. If the poles are reversed, the stimulation threshold will be substantially higher.

The pacing threshold, which is the minimum voltage necessary for pacing stimuli to capture the ventricles consistently, should then be measured (Figure 15.2). It should be less than 1 V, assuming that the pulse generator delivers impulses whose duration is 1 or 2 ms. Some temporary pacemakers allow adjustment of the pulse width: shorter pulse durations lead to a higher threshold and are virtually never indicated for temporary pacing. If the threshold is high, the electrode should be repositioned.

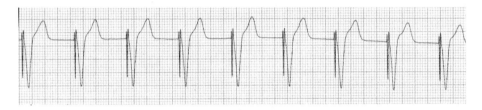

Figure 15.2 Ventricular pacing (lead II). Each pacing stimulus is followed by a ventricular complex. An electrode positioned in the apex of the right ventricle will produce left axis deviation of the paced beats

Sometimes, particularly in an emergency, a pacing threshold or electrode position which is less than optimal has to be accepted. Occasionally a patient may become dependent on the pacemaker, making adjustment of the electrode position hazardous. In these circumstances it may be necessary to insert a second pacing electrode (e.g. via the femoral vein) to cover the period of repositioning.

The stability of the pacing lead should be tested by ensuring that there is consistent pacing during coughing and deep inspiration. During the latter manoeuvre, if there is the correct amount of slack in the lead, there will be a slight curve in its right atrial portion (Figure 15.1E).

To avoid lead displacement, it is essential to securely suture the electrode to the skin at its point of entry.

The pacing threshold often rises to 2–3 V during the first few days after electrode insertion. The threshold should be checked daily and the output set at twice the measured threshold. Battery function and electrical connections should also be checked daily. It is surprising how often the connections between pacemaker and pacing lead, on which a patient's life may depend, are found to be loose or insecure!

Pacing complications

Causes of failure to pace (Figure 15.3) include electrode displacement, myocardial perforation, exit block and a break in either the electrical connections or in the pacing electrode.

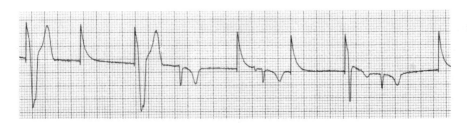

Figure 15.3 Intermittent failure to pace (lead II). Only the first and third pacing stimuli capture the ventricles

Electrode displacement
Electrode displacement may cause intermittent or complete failure to pace. The electrode may fall back into the right atrial cavity and lead to atrial rather than ventricular pacing (Figure 15.4).

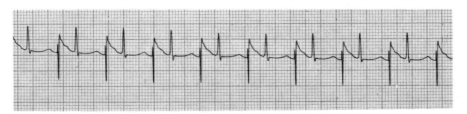

Figure 15.4 Atrial pacing. At the time of this recording, AV conduction was satisfactory so each pacing stimulus was followed by a narrow QRS complex after a PR interval of 0.22 s

Myocardial perforation
Occasionally the electrode tip may perforate the thin right ventricular myocardium. Failure to pace, diaphragmatic stimulation, pericardial friction rub and pericardial pain may result. Cardiac tamponade is extremely rare.

Exit block
Sometimes pacing failure occurs without electrode tip displacement or other cause. In these cases failure is attributed to 'exit block', which is caused by excessive tissue reaction at the junction between electrode tip and endocardium.

Electrical break
A break in the electrical connection or in the electrode itself can be the cause of intermittent or complete pacing failure. In contrast to exit block, no pacing stimuli will appear on the ECG.

Inappropriate inhibition
An occasional cause of pacing failure associated with absent pacing stimuli is external inhibition of a demand pacemaker from electromagnetic waves being emitted from electrical equipment. This problem can be quickly solved by changing the pacemaker to fixed-rate mode.

Failure to sense
Pacemakers are most often used in the 'demand' mode, whereby the pacemaker senses spontaneous cardiac activity and only discharges a stimulus if a spontaneous beat has not occurred within a pre-set period. In some patients, particularly those with myocardial infarction, the signal generated by spontaneous activity may be too small for the pacemaker to sense. As a result, the pacemaker will function in a 'fixed rate' mode and pacing stimuli will be discharged at inappropriate times, and may fall on the T wave of a spontaneous beat (Figure 15.5). This is particularly undesirable in acute myocardial infarction because of the risk of precipitating ventricular fibrillation (Figure 15.6).

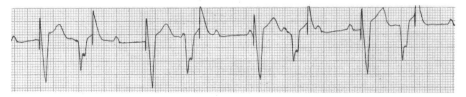

Figure 15.5 Failure to sense in a demand ventricular pacemaker. The first, third, fifth and seventh pacing stimuli capture the ventricles. The second, fourth, sixth and eighth stimuli fall on the T waves of spontaneous ventricular beats

Infection
Infection can occur at the site of entry of a transvenous pacing electrode. Sometimes bacteraemia results: a particularly serious complication if there is valve disease and thus the possibility of endocarditis. Infection will not clear without removal of the pacing electrode. If necessary, a new pacing electrode will have to be inserted at a different site.

AV sequential pacing

Ventricular pacing results in dissociation between atrial and ventricular activity and a consequent reduction in cardiac output of up to one-third.

The atria and ventricles may be paced sequentially enabling the normal sequence of cardiac chamber activation (Figure 15.7). In patients with a low cardiac output, AV sequential pacing can produce an important improvement in cardiac function.

Usually, AV sequential pacing is achieved by passing two leads to the heart: one to the atria and one to the ventricles. The best method of ensuring that an atrial lead is not displaced is to use one with a pre-formed J-shaped terminal portion. A lead of this type can easily be positioned in the right atrial appendage (see Chapter 16).

Temporary transcutaneous and oesophageal pacing

Transcutaneous cardiac pacing was first attempted many years ago but was usually unsuccessful and caused severe discomfort due to skeletal muscle stimulation. Recently,

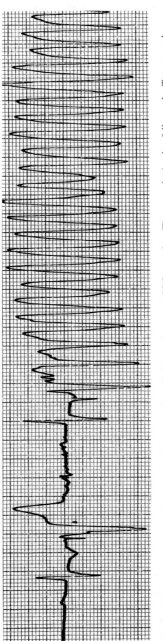

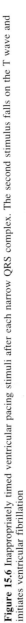

Figure 15.6 Inappropriately timed ventricular pacing stimuli after each narrow QRS complex. The second stimulus falls on the T wave and initiates ventricular fibrillation

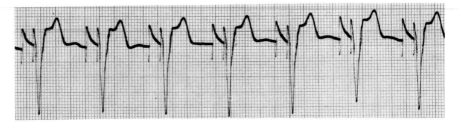

Figure 15.7 AV sequential pacing. Pacing stimuli precede both atrial and ventricular complexes

considerable success with less discomfort has been achieved by using large surface area skin electrodes and stimuli of much longer duration than are used for endocardial stimulation (20–40 ms).

The latest generation of transcutaneous pacemakers function in the demand mode and have a maximum output in the region of 150 mA. One electrode is applied to the front of the chest and the other to the back over the right scapula. Pacing is likely to stimulate the atria at the same time as the ventricles. It is not always possible to ascertain from the ECG that the heart is being stimulated: monitoring of an arterial pulse may be necessary.

With oesophageal pacing, a long impulse duration is necessary (10 ms). Success is more often encountered when stimulating the atria than the ventricles.

As with transvenous pacing, transcutaneous and oesophageal pacing are unlikely to be successful after a prolonged period of cardiac arrest.

Main points

- Indications for temporary transvenous pacing include second- and third-degree AV block due to acute anterior infarction; 'complicated' second- and third-degree AV block due to acute inferior infarction; and recent syncope or near-syncope due to chronic disease of the sinus node or AV junction while awaiting implantation of a long-term pacemaker.
- Subclavian vein puncture is usually the best method of venous access for temporary pacing.
- The pacemaker stimulation threshold, battery function and electrical connections should be checked daily.
- AV sequential pacing improves cardiac output as compared with ventricular pacing.

Long-term cardiac pacing for bradycardias

This subject is discussed in detail to provide a concise account of the practical aspects of pacemaker implantation and the care of patients with pacemakers; often the remit of a cardiac department's more junior members.

An artificial cardiac pacemaker generates electrical stimuli which can initiate myocardial contraction. The stimuli are usually delivered to the heart by transvenous leads or much less commonly via epicardial, oesophageal or transthoracic electrodes.

The first pacemaker was implanted in 1958. Over the following 25 years, rapid progress in technology and an increasing awareness of the benefits of pacing have led to pacemakers being widely used. Patients of all ages, from the newborn to over 100 years old, have been paced: the average age at first implantation is 72 years.

Indications for long-term cardiac pacing

The main reasons for implanting a pacemaker are to relieve symptoms or to improve prognosis. In some patients with asymptomatic impairment of the specialized cardiac conducting system, other factors may also be pertinent such as the need for medication which may cause unwanted bradycardia, or concern in a motor vehicle driver that an accident might result should syncope occur.

Complete atrioventricular block

Syncope

The most common reason for pacemaker implantation is to prevent syncope or near-syncope due to complete AV block. A single episode is a sufficient indication and since the next blackout may cause injury or be fatal, delay should be minimal. Even in patients with a short life expectancy, pacing should be considered if, by preventing syncope, independence may be preserved and serious injury, which may lead to greater demands on medical resources than pacing, may be avoided.

Dyspnoea

Complete heart block can reduce cardiac output and thereby cause exertional dyspnoea and sometimes cardiac failure. Pacing usually improves these problems.

Cerebration

Mental impairment is sometimes attributed to heart block but often does not improve with pacing: if there is doubt, it is best to undertake a trial of temporary pacing.

Prognosis

Without pacing, the prognosis in patients with complete heart block is poor. With an artificial pacemaker, life expectancy closely approaches that of the general population, though those with overt coronary heart disease or with heart failure have a less good outlook. Pacemaker implantation should be considered in asymptomatic patients with complete AV block, particularly when the ventricular rate is 40 beats/minute or less, on purely prognostic grounds.

QRS breadth
Narrow ventricular complexes during complete AV block suggest that interruption in conduction is at AV nodal level and that, in contrast to infranodal block, a subsidiary pacemaker within the bundle of His will discharge reliably at a relatively rapid ventricular rate. However, in practice patients with narrow ventricular complexes during complete heart block may experience syncope and impaired exercise tolerance. In the UK, one-third of patients who receive pacemakers for complete AV block have narrow QRS complexes.

Congenital heart block

Congenital heart block, i.e. complete AV block that is discovered as a neonate or child and is not caused by acquired disease, is widely regarded as benign. However, some patients do develop symptoms or die suddenly. If heart block has caused symptoms then pacing is indicated. In asymptomatic patients the risks of not implanting a pacemaker have to be weighed against the possibility of complications associated with several decades of pacing. Unpaced patients should undergo ambulatory and exercise electrocardiography at regular intervals.

Second-degree AV block

The approach to second-degree AV block is similar to that for complete AV block.

Mobitz II AV block often progresses to complete AV block. A recent study showed that symptoms were commonly associated with Mobitz II AV block and that whereas the prognosis was poor in unpaced patients it was similar to that of the general population in paced patients. This study also refuted the previously held view that Mobitz I AV block is benign in that the incidence of symptoms, prognosis and influence of pacing were the same as for patients with Mobitz II block. This poor outlook does not, however, apply to young people with transient and often nocturnal Wenkebach block which is due to high vagal tone and is benign.

First-degree AV block

First-degree AV block is not itself an indication for cardiac pacing. If a patient presents with first-degree block and syncope or near-syncope it is quite possible that the symptoms are due to transient second- or third-degree AV block, but a pacemaker should not be implanted without proof of this, e.g. by ambulatory electrocardiography.

Bundle branch and fascicular blocks

Bundle branch block

The risk of high-degree AV block developing in an asymptomatic patient with either left or right bundle branch block is very small, and pacing is not indicated. In patients who present with syncope or near-syncope the approach should be the same as for first-degree AV block.

Bifascicular block

In bifascicular block the remaining functioning fascicle may fail to conduct, intermittently or persistently, and cause high-degree AV block. In patients with a good history of Stokes–Adams attacks, pacemaker implantation is indicated to prevent syncope without further investigation. With atypical symptoms, high-degree AV block must be documented first.

In asymptomatic bifascicular block, the chances of progression to complete AV block is in the order of 2% per year and the major determinants of prognosis are the presence of coronary artery or myocardial disease: prophylactic pacing is generally not indicated. Additional first-degree AV block or His bundle electrographic evidence of prolonged infranodal conduction suggest that conduction in the functioning fascicle is also impaired. However, there is no evidence of a higher risk.

AV and bundle branch block after myocardial infarction

AV block due to inferior myocardial infarction usually resolves within a few days and almost always by 3 weeks. When anterior infarction is complicated by high-degree AV block, there is usually extensive myocardial damage and hence the prognosis is poor:

though block may persist it is prudent to ensure that the patient is going to survive before implanting a pacemaker. Thus pacemaker implantation should not be considered unless second- or third-degree AV block is present 3 weeks after myocardial infarction.

When a patient is admitted to hospital with heart block, there is often an unnecessary delay before referral for long-term pacing while myocardial infarction is excluded. Unless the patient has experienced typical cardiac pain or there are obvious ECG changes of recent infarction, AV block has probably not been caused by acute infarction.

Bifascicular block persisting after acute anterior infarction complicated by AV block raises the possibility that complete AV block might recur. Intermittent heart block has been demonstrated to occur in some patients with post-infarction bifascicular block and may necessitate pacing. However, prophylactic pacing does not reduce mortality.

Sick sinus syndrome

Syncope

Sick sinus syndrome accounts for one-quarter of pacemaker implantations. Pacing is indicated when syncope or near-syncope are caused. It should be remembered that sinus bradycardia and pauses in sinus node activity for up to 2 s, particularly if nocturnal, can be physiological.

Bradycardia-tachycardia syndrome

In patients with the bradycardia-tachycardia syndrome, pacing may be required to avoid severe bradycardia caused by anti-arrhythmic drugs. Sometimes tachyarrhythmias which start during bradycardia will be prevented by atrial pacing.

Prognosis

Pacing for sick sinus syndrome does not improve prognosis and is not usually indicated in asymptomatic patients. However, pauses in cardiac activity for several seconds might be considered an indication for pacing in those who operate machinery, including a motor car, to avoid an accident should syncope occur.

Hypersensitive carotid sinus and malignant vasovagal syndromes

Pacing will improve symptoms in these syndromes, provided that there is a significant cardio-inhibitory component (Chapter 10).

Hypertrophic obstructive cardiomyopathy

Recently, dual chambered pacing has been shown to reduce symptoms and left ventricular outflow tract gradient in patients with hypertrophic obstructive cardiomyopathy during sinus rhythm.

Pacing modes

The first generation of pacemakers functioned in a fixed-rate mode: the pacemaker stimulated the ventricles regularly, usually at 70 beats/minute, irrespective of any spontaneous cardiac activity (Figure 16.1). Competition with a spontaneous rhythm could

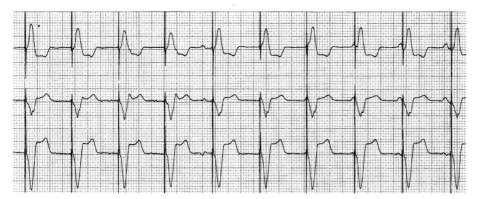

Figure 16.1 Fixed-rate ventricular pacing (leads I, II, III). A large pacing stimulus precedes each ventricular complex

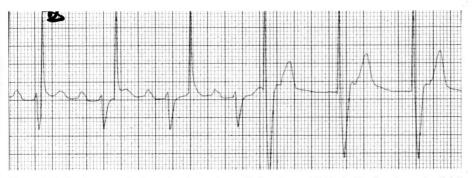

Figure 16.2 Fixed-rate ventricular pacing in a patient with first-degree AV block. The first three stimuli fall during the refractory period and are ineffective. The fourth causes a premature contraction

cause irregular palpitation (Figure 16.2), and stimulation during ventricular repolarization could possibly initiate ventricular fibrillation.

Subsequent developments enabled sensing of spontaneous activity via the stimulating lead to facilitate demand pacing: a sensed event resets the timing of delivery of the next pacemaker stimulus to avoid competition with spontaneous activity (Figure 16.3).

With the advent of reliable transvenous atrial pacing leads it became straightforward to pace and sense in the atrium as well as the ventricle, thus allowing both atrial and

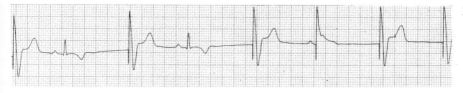

Figure 16.3 Demand ventricular pacemaker. The pacemaker is inhibited by the sinus beats (second and fourth complexes). The sixth complex is a fusion beat. A P wave can be seen to precede the pacing stimulus. By chance, a sinus impulse has arisen at the instant when the pacemaker was set to discharge and the ventricles have been activated by both stimulus impulse and pacemaker. Fusion beats should not be confused with failure to pace

ventricular 'single chamber' pacing and also 'dual chamber' pacing whereby stimulation and/or sensing can take place at both atrial and ventricular levels. These developments have permitted a more physiological approach to cardiac stimulation.

Pacing system code

A five letter code is widely used to describe the various pacing modes; the first three characters are the most important.

The first character identifies the chamber or chambers that are paced: 'A' for atrium, 'V' for ventricle and 'D' (for double) if both atrium and ventricle can be stimulated.

The second character indicates the chamber or chambers whose activity is sensed: in addition to the use of 'A', 'V' and 'D', 'O' indicates that the pacemaker is insensitive.

The third character denotes the response to the sensed information: 'I' indicates that pacemaker output is inhibited by a sensed event, 'T' that stimulation is triggered by a sensed event and 'D' that ventricular sensed events inhibit pacemaker output while atrial sensed events trigger ventricular stimulation; 'O' indicates that there is no response to sensed events.

A fourth character, 'R', is used if there is a rate responsive facility whereby the pacing rate is modulated by a sensor that detects a physiological variable such as activity or respiration.

The fifth character relates to anti-tachycardia functions: 'O', none; 'P', anti-tachycardia pacing (low-energy stimulation); 'S', shock (i.e. cardioversion or defibrillation); and 'D', both anti-tachycardia pacing and shock.

Single chamber pacing

Ventricular demand pacing

In the absence of spontaneous ventricular activity, a ventricular demand pacemaker, like a fixed-rate unit, delivers stimuli to the ventricles at a regular rate. However, if spontaneous activity is sensed via the ventricular lead, the timing of delivery of the next pacemaker output is reset to avoid competition.

In ventricular inhibited (VVI) pacemakers a sensed event terminates the current stimulation cycle, thus inhibiting pacemaker output, and starts a new cycle (Figure 16.3). In contrast, a sensed event during the less commonly used mode of ventricular triggered (VVT) pacing immediately triggers delivery of a pacing stimulus which will consequently fall during the myocardial refractory period and will thus be ineffective: the subsequent cycle will then start from delivery of the triggered impulsive (Figure 16.4).

The pacemaker is rendered insensitive immediately after a paced or sensed event for an interval which approximates the duration of myocardial activation and recovery to prevent

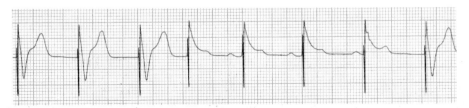

Figure 16.4 Ventricular triggered pacemaker. After the first three paced beats there is sinus rhythm. A pacing stimulus is discharged immediately after the onset of the QRS complex in these beats

sensing the ventricular electrogram which is produced by the event; this interval (250–300 ms) is referred to as the refractory period.

Ventricular demand pacing is a commonly employed mode but its use is diminishing now its disadvantages – the inabilities to facilitate the normal sequence of cardiac chamber activation and to provide a chronotropic response to exercise – are widely appreciated (see below).

Indisputable indications for ventricular demand pacing include bradycardia associated with persistent atrial fibrillation, second- and third-degree AV block in patients who are limited by impaired cerebral or locomotor function and patients with infrequent bradycardia in whom the pacemaker is mainly on 'stand-by'.

Atrial demand pacing

The timing cycles of atrial inhibited (AAI) and the less commonly used atrial triggered (AAT) modes are the same as for ventricular demand pacing, as described above (Figure 16.5). With atrial pacing, the refractory period is usually longer to avoid sensing the 'far field' ventricular electrogram which may be sensed via the atrial lead and which may inappropriately inhibit the pacemaker.

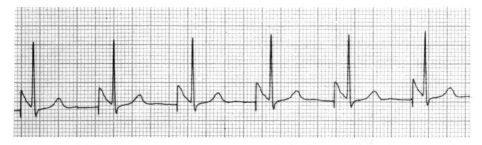

Figure 16.5 Atrial pacing. A pacing stimulus precedes each P wave.

Atrial pacing is indicated for treatment of the sick sinus syndrome unless AV conduction is impaired. By stimulating the atria rather than the ventricles, the normal sequence of cardiac chamber activation is maintained, loss of which can reduce cardiac output by up to one-third.

Sick sinus syndrome can be associated with impaired AV conduction. However, if there is no evidence of it at the time of pacemaker implantation the development of impaired AV conduction is uncommon. If atrial pacing at a rate of 120 beats/minute causes second-degree AV block or if there is bifascicular or bundle branch block, dual chamber pacing is indicated.

Dual chamber pacing

AV sequential pacing

In AV sequential (DVI) pacing the atria are stimulated first and then, after a delay which approximates the normal PR interval, the ventricles are stimulated (Figure 16.6). The pacemaker is inhibited by spontaneous ventricular activity but no sensing occurs in the atrium. As with other dual chamber modes, both atrial and ventricular electrodes are required.

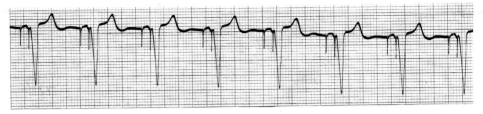

Figure 16.6 AV sequential (DVI) pacing. Pacing stimuli precede both atrial and ventricular complexes

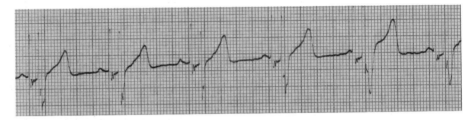

Figure 16.7 DVI pacing: fusion beats

There are non-committed and committed versions of AV sequential pacing. With the former, a sensed ventricular event during the interval between atrial and ventricular stimulation will inhibit delivery of the ventricular stimulus. With the latter, ventricular stimulation will always follow the atrial stimulus.

Fusion beats (Figure 16.7) are commonly seen during DVI pacing and are sometimes misinterpreted as pacemaker malfunction: whereas the pacemaker is inhibited by an event sensed in the ventricles, the first chamber to be stimulated is the atrium. Pacemaker output may therefore occur at the same time as spontaneous atrial activation because its resultant ventricular depolarization has not yet occurred.

More recently, the mode of DDI pacing has been introduced. Sensing occurs at atrial as well as ventricular levels but unlike DDD pacing (see below), sensed atrial events do not trigger ventricular stimulation. Thus this mode cannot facilitate endless loop tachycardia, a complication of dual chamber pacing which is described below.

The main indications for DVI and DDI pacing are sick sinus syndrome associated with impaired AV conduction and carotid sinus and malignant vasovagal syndromes.

Atrial synchronized ventricular pacing

In this mode, ventricular stimulation is triggered by a sensed atrial event after an interval similar to the normal PR interval (Figure 16.8). It thereby maintains the normal sequence

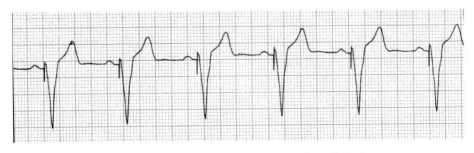

Figure 16.8 Atrial synchronized pacing. Each P wave triggers a paced ventricular beat

of cardiac chamber activation and permits a chronotropic response to exercise, provided that sinus node function is normal.

If an atrial event is not sensed, ventricular stimulation continues at a fixed cycle length – otherwise atrial standstill might lead to ventricular asystole. To avoid atrial tachycardia or fibrillation triggering inappropriately fast ventricular pacing rates, there is an atrial refractory interval: the atrial channel is rendered insensitive during the AV delay and for a period after ventricular stimulation. Sensed atrial activity at a cycle length shorter than this period will not trigger ventricular stimulation.

The upper rate at which atrial activity will trigger ventricular output is determined by the 'total atrial refractory period' which consists of the AV delay plus the post-ventricular stimulus refractory period. For example, if the AV delay is 125 ms and the atrial refractory period is 250 ms, the upper rate limit will be 60 000/375 = 160 beats/minute.

In earlier years, sensing only took place in the atrium and pacing only occurred in the ventricle (VAT). Thus ventricular ectopic beats or rhythms faster than the sinus node rate would not inhibit ventricular output. Subsequently, VDD pacing was introduced whereby sensing takes place in the ventricles as well, so that spontaneous ventricular activity will inhibit the pacemaker (Figure 16.9).

Atrial synchronized ventricular pacing is indicated in second- and third-degree AV block when sinus node function is normal. It is contraindicated in sick sinus syndrome or when there are atrial tachyarrhythmias.

'Endless loop tachycardia'

If a ventricular stimulus is conducted retrogradely to the atria via either the AV junction or, if present, an accessory AV pathway, and the timing of the resultant atrial activation is outside the pacemaker's atrial refractory period, it will trigger ventricular stimulation and hence initiate an 'endless loop tachycardia' (Figure 16.10), also referred to as 'pacemaker-mediated tachycardia'. Ventriculoatrial conduction is present in approximately two-thirds of patients with sick sinus syndrome and one-fifth of those with complete AV block. Endless loop tachycardia can usually be prevented by prolongation of the atrial refractory period but at the expense of reduction of the upper rate limit for ventricular stimulation. Endless loop tachycardia can be avoided in 90% of patients by setting the AV delay to 125 ms and the post-ventricular atrial refractory period to 300 ms.

Most pacemakers can detect endless loop tachycardia and interrupt it: for example, by prolonging the atrial refractory period for one cycle.

AV universal pacing

In this mode (DDD), both sensing and pacing can take place at atrial and ventricular levels. Universal pacing allows the pacemaker to function in atrial demand (AAI), AV sequential (DVI, DDI) or atrial synchronized (VDD) modes depending on the spontaneous heart rhythm (Figure 16.11).

If there is sinus bradycardia, it functions as an atrial demand pacemaker. If there is impaired AV conduction, ventricular pacing is triggered by either spontaneous atrial activity or by delivery of an atrial stimulus. When sinus node function is normal, it functions in the atrial synchronized mode, thus providing a chronotropic response to exercise. The pacemaker is inhibited by both atrial and ventricular ectopic beats. Endless loop tachycardia may occur if there is retrograde AV conduction.

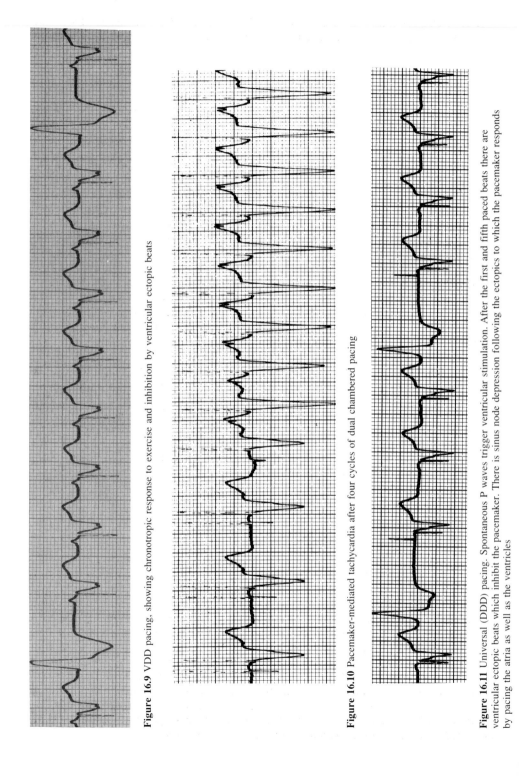

Figure 16.9 VDD pacing, showing chronotropic response to exercise and inhibition by ventricular ectopic beats

Figure 16.10 Pacemaker-mediated tachycardia after four cycles of dual chambered pacing

Figure 16.11 Universal (DDD) pacing. Spontaneous P waves trigger ventricular stimulation. After the first and fifth paced beats there are ventricular ectopic beats which inhibit the pacemaker. There is sinus node depression following the ectopics to which the pacemaker responds by pacing the atria as well as the ventricles

DDD pacing is indicated in second- and third-degree AV block and in sinus node dysfunction. Atrial tachyarrhythmias are a contraindication.

'Physiological pacing'

Physiological pacing systems facilitate a chronotropic response to exercise by maintaining atrioventricular synchronization as the sinus node rate varies and/or by a rate adaptive mechanism.

Atrial synchronized ventricular pacing

This mode which both maintains AV synchronization and facilitates a chronotropic response has been shown to increase cardiac output at rest and during exercise as compared with ventricular pacing. Exercise capacity has been measured on a double-blind basis during ventricular pacing at 70 beats/minute and during atrial synchronized ventricular pacing. The latter mode has been demonstrated to increase maximal exercise capacity by approximately 30%. However, individual patients varied in the degree by which they benefited: in a few there was little improvement whereas in a many there was a dramatic increase. Neither age nor cause of heart block predicted the amount of benefit. It used to be thought that 'physiological' pacing was of greatest value to patients with poor ventricular function. This is not the case; indeed, patients with high venous pressures may not benefit.

Atrial synchronized pacing improves parameters in addition to maximal exercise tolerance. Shortness of breadth, dizziness and palpitation are less frequent whereas fixed rate pacing tends to impair the normal blood pressure response to exercise and leads to a higher respiratory rate and perceived exertion during submaximal exercise. The advantages of atrial synchronized pacing have been shown to be maintained long term.

There are limitations to atrial synchronized ventricular pacing. First, normal or at least near-normal sinus node activity is required. Secondly, the ventricular stimulation rate may increase in response to an atrial tachyarrhythmia. Thirdly, an atrial as well as a ventricular pacing lead is required.

Rate response systems

Several pacing systems are available that can facilitate a chronotropic response independent of atrial activity: a change in stimulation rate is achieved in response to a parameter that alters with exercise. In contrast to atrial synchronized pacing, normal sinus node activity is not required.

According to the pacemaker code, a ventricular demand and a dual chambered pacemaker with a rate response facility are termed VVIR and DDDR, respectively.

In terms of exercise capacity, the ability to increase heart rate is far more important than maintaining atrioventricular synchronization. This has been demonstrated by measuring exercise tolerance during three pacing modes: fixed rate, atrial synchronized, and ventricular pacing at a rate equal to but not synchronized with atrial activity. Both the latter forms of chronotropic pacing increased exercise performance to a similar degree as compared with fixed rate pacing. Thus rate response ventricular pacemakers can enable an enhanced exercise tolerance without the need for an atrial lead.

Activity sensor

Vibration resulting from physical activity is sensed by a piezoelectric crystal. The stimulation rate increases in parallel with the level of sensed vibration. The system has been criticized because it is not truly physiological. For example, the same levels of vibration and hence the same heart rate will be generated by ascending and descending a flight of stairs, though less work is required for the latter. However, in contrast to systems using other sensors, a very prompt chronotropic response to exercise is achieved.

Evoked QT response

Though it has been known for many years that the QT interval decreases with increasing heart rate, it has only recently been appreciated that sympathetic nervous system activity is a major independent determinant of QT interval duration: QT interval shortens during exercise even during fixed-rate pacing. The pacemaker senses, via a conventional ventricular pacing electrode, the interval between pacing stimulus and apex of the evoked T wave: a decrease in the interval leads to an increase in stimulation rate.

Since this system responds to sympathetic nervous system activity, it will increase the heart rate in response to emotion as well as exertion.

Respiration

There is a close relation between minute volume and heart rate. The system's discharge rate is governed by changes in intravascular impedance, a measure of respiratory minute volume, which is monitored by means of a conventional bipolar pacing lead.

Blood temperature

Skeletal muscle activity generates heat which is transferred to the blood. There is a relation between level of exercise and right ventricular blood temperature. One problem, however, is that there is a latency in the system due to the delay of 1 or 2 minutes before blood temperature rises after the start of exercise.

Other sensors

Other parameters such as oxygen saturation and right ventricular pressure are being investigated for use in rate response pacing. Information on long-term reliability of sensors is not yet available. Rate response systems that can use a conventional lead have practical advantages over systems that require a lead incorporating a specialized sensor.

Multisensor pacing

Dual chamber pacemakers are now available which in addition to sensing atrial activity will respond to parameters related to exercise such as activity or QT interval (DDDR). Thus, normal AV synchrony can be maintained and a chronotropic response to exercise can be provided even if sinus node function is impaired or if an intermittent atrial arrhythmia occurs.

Some newer pacing systems incorporate not one but two types of physiological sensor so that the limitations of each system can be minimized. For example, an activity sensor to provide a prompt response and a QT sensor to ensure the rate response is proportional to the workload.

'Pacemaker syndrome'

It is at rest that the disadvantage of loss of AV synchrony caused by ventricular pacing may become apparent. Atrial contraction may occur against closed mitral and tricuspid

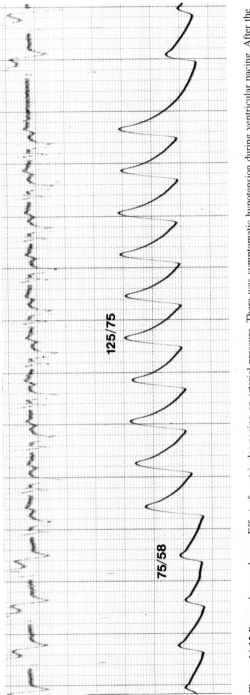
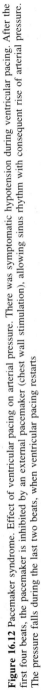

Figure 16.12 Pacemaker syndrome. Effect of ventricular pacing on arterial pressure. There was symptomatic hypotension during ventricular pacing. After the first four beats, the pacemaker is inhibited by an external pacemaker (chest wall stimulation), allowing sinus rhythm with consequent rise of arterial pressure. The pressure falls during the last two beats, when ventricular pacing restarts

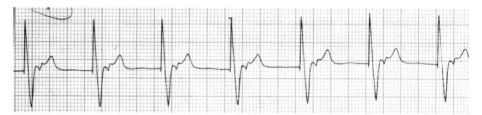

Figure 16.13 Ventricular pacing with retrograde activation (lead II). Each ventricular complex is followed by an inverted P wave

valves. Atrial pressure will rise and impede venous return so that during the next diastolic period the ventricles will be underfilled with resultant reduction in stroke volume. Loss of properly timed atrial systole reduces cardiac output by up to one-third and may cause hypotension: near-syncope and syncope can result (Figure 16.12). Ventriculoatrial conduction (Figure 16.13) causes even greater haemodynamic upset: the resultant atrial distension may initiate a reflex vasodepressor effect.

Hypotension is likely to be more marked whilst standing. It is most severe during the first few seconds of ventricular pacing, before vasoconstrictor compensatory mechanisms can come into play, so ventricular pacing is particularly unsuitable for patients who are mainly in sinus rhythm but who often develop bradycardia at a rate less than the cycle length of the ventricular pacemaker, i.e. those with sick sinus or carotid sinus syndromes. This has been demonstrated by recording ambulatory blood pressure in patients with ventricular demand pacemakers. The onset of ventricular pacing was followed by hypotension which was greater in those who had complained of syncope and near-syncope. Atrioventricular sequential pacing or, when AV conduction is not impaired, atrial pacing will avoid these problems.

Pacemaker hardware

Pulse generator

A pulse generator consists of a power source together with electronic circuits to control the timing and characteristics of the impulses that it generates.

In the past, several power sources have been used including mercury-zinc cells, rechargeable nickel-cadmium cells and nuclear energy. Now, lithium iodide cells are used almost exclusively. Lithium pacemakers have a lifespan of 4–15 years and a predictable, progressive discharge behaviour. They are contained in a hermetically sealed titanium can, 35–50 g in weight, and generally have a maximum diameter of no more than 50 mm and a thickness of as little as 6 mm.

Pacemaker leads

Stimuli produced by the pulse generator are conducted to the heart via a lead which consists of an insulated wire with an electrode at its tip which is attached to the heart.

Transvenous leads are used in over 95% of pacemaker implantations. A modern lead consists of a multifilar, helically coiled wire which is insulated by a material that does not cause tissue reaction or thrombosis: silicone rubber or polyurethane.

At the lead tip is the cathode which is composed of an inert material such as platinum-iridium, elgiloy, steel or vitreous carbon. For effective stimulation, this must be securely and closely attached to the endocardium. If fibrous tissue, which is non-excitable, develops between cathode and endocardium the amount of energy required to stimulate the heart will increase and may exceed the output capability of the pacemaker.

To achieve a low threshold for stimulation and secure endocardial attachment, several 'fixation devices' have been employed. 'Passive' fixation devices include tines, flanges or fins positioned proximal to the lead tip which can become entrapped in the myocardial trabeculae. 'Active' devices include an electrode in the shape of a helix which by rotation of the lead can be wound around a trabeculum, and a retractable metal screw which can be screwed into the endo-myocardium. 'Porous' metal or carbon electrodes are now widely used: the surface of the cathode consists of many microscopic pores which promote rapid tissue ingrowth and hence very secure fixation. Movement between electrode and endocardium and thus generation of fibrous tissue is minimized. One type of electrode elutes dexamethasone to minimize local tissue reaction and hence stimulation threshold.

Attachment of atrial leads was impracticable until the advent of fixation devices. The distal portion of atrial leads are often 'J'-shaped to facilitate positioning in the right atrial appendage.

The amount of energy required to stimulate the heart is related to the surface area of the cathode. Nowadays, low surface area electrodes are used ($6-12 \, mm^2$).

Leads that are sewn on to the epicardium or screwed into the myocardium necessitate thoracotomy and are now, with the advent of reliable transvenous leads, rarely used unless pacemaker implantation is undertaken at the time of open heart surgery; or venous thrombosis or tricuspid valve prosthesis preclude a transvenous approach.

Unipolar versus bipolar pacing

In unipolar pacing the anode is remote from the heart; usually the metal can containing the pulse generator. In bipolar pacing, both anode and cathode are within the cardiac chamber to be paced, the anode positioned along the lead near to its cathodal tip. A commonly held view is that an electrogram sensed by a unipolar lead is larger than that from a bipolar lead. There is in fact usually no difference between bipolar and unipolar electrograms or stimulation thresholds.

Bipolar pacing has the advantage that inappropriate sensing of electromagnetic interference and skeletal muscle electromyograms is much less likely, as is extracardiac stimulation. Reasons for favouring unipolar pacing are that there is greater experience with unipolar leads, that leads have in the past been thinner and that surface ECG unipolar pacemaker stimuli are larger, enabling ECG interpretation.

Costs

In the UK, the current (1992) approximate costs of a pulse generator plus leads for single chamber, programmable single chamber and dual chambered pacing systems are £600, £800 and £1500, respectively.

Pacemaker implantation

Facilities for fluoroscopy, ECG monitoring and cardiopulmonary resuscitation are required. The procedure is usually carried out under local anaesthesia and takes 15–45 minutes.

Subclavian approach

The subclavian approach is now widely used and is especially useful if more than one lead is to be inserted. The pacemaker lead(s) are introduced via infraclavicular subclavian vein puncture and are connected to the pulse generator which is implanted in a subcutaneous pocket fashioned over pectoralis major.

An incision is made 2 cm below the junction of the middle and inner thirds of the clavicle and is extended in a lateral and usually inferior direction for approximately 7 cm. A subcutaneous pocket large enough to accommodate the pulse generator is created by blunt dissection.

Puncture of the subclavian vein is easier if the vein is distended: a slight head-down position will help. A needle is introduced just below the inferior border of the clavicle at the junction of its middle and inner thirds and directed towards the sternoclavicular joint so that it passes behind the posterior surface of the clavicle. As the needle punctures the vein, venous blood will be aspirated easily: only a trickle suggests that the needle is not in the vein. Aspiration of air or bright pulsatile blood indicate puncture of the pleura or subclavian artery, respectively. If the patient has a 'deep' chest, and particularly if the clavicle bows anteriorly, it may be necessary to introduce the needle a little more laterally and to point it slightly posteriorly.

Cannulation of the vein is then achieved by introducing a flexible guide wire, preferably with a J-shaped tip, through the needle. Resistance to its passage indicates that the wire is not in the vein. The wire is passed into the superior vena cava and its position checked by fluoroscopy. The needle is then withdrawn and a sheath within which is a vessel dilator is passed over the wire into the vein. The guide wire and dilator are then removed and the pacing lead inserted into the sheath. If it is planned to introduce a second pacing lead, then the guide wire can be left in place to permit introduction of a second introducer and sheath. 'Peel-away' sheaths are used so that their removal is not prevented by the connector at the proximal end of the lead.

Cephalic vein approach

An alternative to subclavian vein puncture is to cut down onto the cephalic vein in the deltopectoral groove. This approach avoids the risks of subclavian vein puncture but the vein may not be big enough to accommodate two leads and sometimes is even too small for one lead.

Occasionally, a cut-down technique is used with the jugular, axillary or pectoral veins.

Positioning of a ventricular lead

To facilitate manipulation of a long-term pacing lead, which is very flexible, a wire stylet is passed down the centre of the lead. Bending the distal part of the stylet or slight withdrawal will often aid positioning.

The lead is passed into the right atrium (see Figure 15.1). Sometimes the lead can then be directly advanced through the tricuspid valve to the right ventricular apex. More often, it is necessary to form a loop in the atrium by impinging the lead tip on the atrial wall and then advancing the lead a little further. By rotating the lead its tip can then be positioned near the tricuspid valve. Slight withdrawal of the lead will allow it to 'flick' through the valve into the ventricle. Ventricular ectopic beats are usually provoked as the valve is crossed. If these do not occur then the coronary sinus may have been entered. Entry into the ventricle can be confirmed by advancing the lead into the pulmonary artery. Once in the right ventricle, the lead tip is positioned in or near the ventricular apex by a process of lead rotation, advancement and withdrawal. A stable position should be ensured by checking for continuous pacing and for absence of excessive lead tip movement during deep inspiration and coughing. Once a satisfactory position has been achieved both in terms of stability and measurements (see below), it is very important that the lead is secured by placing a short length of rubber sleeve around it near its point of entry into the vein and fixing it to the underlying muscle with a non-adsorbable suture.

Positioning of an atrial lead

The right atrial appendage is the usual site for atrial pacing. If necessary, atrial pacing may be performed by using a 'screw-in' lead to pace from the septal or free right atrial walls.

For pacing the right atrial appendage, a lead with a J-shaped terminal portion is usually used. First, using a straight stylet the lead tip is straightened and advanced to the mid-right atrium. The lead is then rotated so that its tip is near the tricuspid valve. Partial withdrawal of the stylet causes the lead to assume its J shape and slight withdrawal of the lead itself allows the lead tip to enter the appendage. A straight lead may be positioned in the appendage by use of a stylet whose terminal 5–7 cm have been shaped into a tight 'J'.

Correct positioning will be demonstrated by the lead tip moving from side to side with atrial systole. Lateral screening should demonstrate that the lead is pointing anteriorly. Lead stability should be confirmed by twisting the lead 45° in either direction: the lead tip should not turn. It is important that there is the correct amount of slack in the lead: during inspiration the angle between the two limbs of the J should not exceed 80°.

Measurement of stimulation and sensing thresholds

Low stimulation and sensing thresholds are essential for satisfactory long-term pacing. High thresholds suggest that the cathode is not in close apposition to excitable tissue. Thresholds rise after pacemaker implantation, usually peaking 3 weeks to 3 months after surgery. If they become high they may exceed the stimulation and sensing capabilities of the pulse generator.

Thresholds are usually measured with a commercially produced pacing systems analyser. It is preferable to match the analyser with the generator to be implanted so that they have similar impulse generating and sensing circuits. The same unipolar or bipolar electrode configuration should be used as is planned to use with the implanted system.

Stimulation threshold

The stimulation threshold is the smallest electrical stimulus (delivered by the cathode outside the ventricular effective and relative refractory periods) which will consistently activate the myocardium.

To measure the stimulation threshold, the analyser is set to deliver impulses at 70 beats/ minute (or if there is no bradycardia at the time, 10 beats/minute in excess of the spontaneous rate) with an impulse duration similar to that which the implanted pulse generator will deliver (often 0.5 ms) and a voltage output of 5 V. The threshold is then established by progressively reducing the output until failure of capture occurs: if the patient has no spontaneous rhythm, pacemaker output will have to be promptly increased to avoid asystole. At a pulse duration of 0.5 ms, a voltage threshold of less than 1 V is satisfactory: usually the threshold will be in the region of 0.5 V. If the stimulation threshold is measured by progressively increasing the output from a subthreshold level, it will be found to be slightly higher: the Wedensky phenomenon.

The longer the duration of the pacing stimulus the more energy is delivered and hence the lower is the stimulation threshold. However, the relationship is not linear: the range of efficient impulse duration, in terms of energy consumption, is 0.25–1.0 ms.

Sensing threshold

To ensure satisfactory sensing it is important that the intracardiac electrogram resulting from spontaneous activity of the cardiac chamber to be paced is of sufficient amplitude. It is usually measured with a pacing systems analyser. Ventricular and atrial electrograms should be greater than 4 mV and 2 mV, respectively. In 'borderline' cases the slew rate, i.e. the rate of change of signal voltage, is also important: low rates may result in failure to sense.

Lead impedance

The pacing systems analyser can also be used to measure lead impedance which is a measure of resistance to flow of current in the lead. It varies with lead type but is usually in the order of 400–800 Ω.

A low impedance suggests a break in insulation and hence leakage of current, whereas a high impedance points to lead fracture.

Complications of pacemaker implantation

Mild bruising is not uncommon but, occasionally, poor haemostasis will result in a haematoma which if tense should be evacuated.

Infection should occur in less than 1% of implantations and is virtually always staphyloccocal. Unless it is only superficial, explantation will usually be required even if antibiotics appear to help initially. Ideally, the pacing lead(s) should be removed. However, fixation devices can make removal difficult and introduce the risk of tamponade. Use of a special lead extraction device may be effective. Sometimes it is necessary to resort to thoracotomy. Alternatively, the lead can be shortened so that it no longer lies in the infected area, capping its proximal end and fixing it with a suture, but there is a risk of persistent infection and bacteraemia.

Prophylactic antibiotics are widely used but there is little evidence that they are of value.

Erosion is a late complication but is often a consequence of implantation technique. Factors that predispose to erosion include creation of a pacemaker pocket which is too tight or too superficial, a very thin patient, and use of a generator with sharp corners. The skin will be found to be thinned around the site of erosion. Infection is often present but it is secondary to erosion. If 'threatened' erosion is detected the generator may be re-sited but if the skin is broken explantation will be necessary.

Lead displacement was once a common problem but with modern leads it occurs in less than 1% of implantations: it necessitates re-operation.

Complications of attempted subclavian vein puncture are infrequent: they include pneumothorax, haemothorax, air embolism, brachial plexus damage and puncture of the subclavian artery.

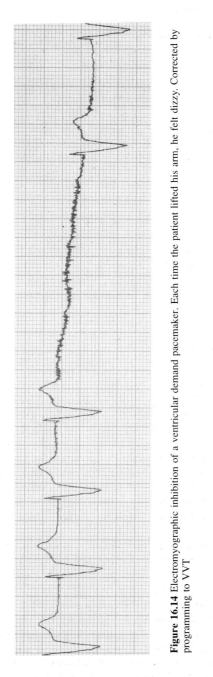

Figure 16.14 Electromyographic inhibition of a ventricular demand pacemaker. Each time the patient lifted his arm, he felt dizzy. Corrected by programming to VVT

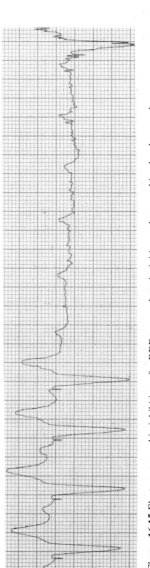

Figure 16.15 Electromyographic inhibition of a DDD pacemaker. Activities such as washing hands caused near-syncope. Corrected by decreasing pacemaker sensitivity

Fashioning of a generator pocket which is too large may allow spontaneous or intentional repeated rotation of the pulse generator which can cause dislodgement or fracture of the pacing lead: the 'twiddler's syndrome'.

Complications related to pulse generator

Electromyographic interference

This common problem is virtually confined to unipolar pacing systems. Myopotentials generated from the underlying muscle are sensed by the pacemaker as spontaneous cardiac activity (Figures 16.14 and 16.15). In systems where sensed events inhibit output, inappropriate cessation of pacing will occur. Short periods of electromyographic inhibition are common and usually asymptomatic. Longer periods may cause syncope and necessitate re-operation, or in programmable pacemakers (see below), adjustment to sensitivity, pacing mode or polarity.

Susceptibility to electromyographic inhibition can be demonstrated by asking the patient to extend his arms and then press his hands firmly together. Inhibition is only significant if it lasts for several seconds, particularly if the patient's symptoms are reproduced.

Muscle stimulation

This complication is also related to unipolar pacing. It is a consequence of the pacemaker can being the anode: stimulation of the underlying pectoral muscle occurs. Most unipolar pacemakers now have an insulating covering applied to the back and sides of the pacemaker so that the only anodal contact is with the subcutaneous tissues.

Generator failure

Premature generator failure does occur occasionally.

Complications related to pacing lead

Exit block

The development of excessive fibrous tissue, which is non-excitable, around the cathode may increase the stimulation threshold to a level higher than the pacemaker's output. The result will be intermittent or persistent failure to pace without evidence of lead displacement (Figure 16.16). Exit block is most likely to occur in the first 3 weeks to 3 months after implantation when stimulation threshold is at its highest. Sometimes exit block is transient, otherwise lead repositioning will be required unless generator output can be increased by reprogramming (see below). Modern leads with low surface area, porous surfaced electrodes and positive fixation devices rarely give rise to this complication.

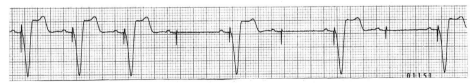
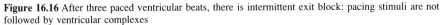

Figure 16.16 After three paced ventricular beats, there is intermittent exit block: pacing stimuli are not followed by ventricular complexes

Lead fracture

With modern leads, fracture is rare. If it does occur it is usually at the point where the lead enters the venous system, at the site of a fixation suture or wherever there is excessive angulation of the lead. Lead fracture will cause intermittent or persistent failure to pace and sense. Lead fracture can often be detected radiographically but should not be confused with 'pseudofracture': the pressure of a tight ligature directly applied to the lead may compress the insulation and spread the coils of wire inside without interfering with lead function.

Insulation breakdown

This will allow leakage of current, which may cause stimulation of adjacent muscles, and hence premature battery depletion. A tight ligature anchoring the lead without use of a rubber sleeve is the commonest cause. Some types of polyurethane insulation are prone to this problem.

Phrenic nerve and diaphragmatic stimulation

The phrenic nerve or diaphragm can sometimes be stimulated through the intervening thin myocardial walls by atrial and ventricular leads, respectively. Lead repositioning will be required unless, in programmable pacemakers, cessation of extra-cardiac stimulation can be achieved by output reduction.

Venous thrombosis

Clinically apparent subclavian vein thrombosis is rare and pulmonary embolism even rarer. Anticoagulant therapy is indicated. Angiographic studies have reported that asymptomatic venous thrombosis is not infrequent.

Pacemaker programmability

A programmable pacemaker can be non-invasively adjusted in one or more of its functions by radiofrequency signals emitted from an external programming device. Programmability enables achievement of optimal pacemaker function for the individual patient and can also be used in the diagnosis and treatment of certain pacemaker complications: it reduces the need for pacemaker re-operation and some authorities regard their use as mandatory.

Simple programmable pacemakers permit alteration to rate and output. In multi-programmable pacemakers a wide variety of parameters can be adjusted. These are listed below, together with typical options:

1. Lower rate limit (30–150 beats/minute).
2. Output (2.5–5.0 V or 1–12 mA).
3. Sensitivity (0.5–8 mV).
4. Pacing mode (e.g. inhibited, triggered or rate response).
5. Refractory period (200–500 ms).
6. Pacing polarity (uni- or bipolar).
7. AV delay (0–250 ms) (for dual chamber pacemakers).
8. Upper rate limits (100–180 beats/minute) (for dual chamber and rate response pacemakers).

Recently, software-based pacemakers have been introduced. Many functions are controlled by a microcomputer within the pacemaker which can be externally programmed: functions can be modified and new developments incorporated that had not even been anticipated at the time of implantation.

Some examples of the advantages of programmability are discussed below.

In patients who are mainly in sinus rhythm, reduction of the stand-by rate will allow sinus rhythm to be maintained for longer periods and will therefore help to avoid the haemodynamic disadvantages of ventricular pacing. Reduction of stimulation rate may occasionally help in the management of angina. Sometimes an increase in rate is helpful in the treatment of cardiac failure or arrhythmias.

Usually, the stimulation threshold is a lot lower than the maximum output of a pacemaker; a reduction in output will prolong battery life. At regular intervals, the threshold can be measured by progressive reduction in output and then the output programmed to the threshold value plus a safety margin. Extracardiac stimulation can often be stopped by reduction in output without approaching the threshold level. Some pacemakers have a high output facility (e.g. ability to increase output from 5 to 10 V): use of this may avoid the need for re-operation should exit block, which may be a temporary problem, occur.

Increase in sensitivity of the amplifier circuits may help with undersensing whereas inappropriate sensing of T waves or after-potentials may be dealt with by reduction in sensitivity or prolongation of refractory period.

Reduction in sensitivity may prevent electromyographic inhibition. Alternatively, reprogramming from inhibited to triggered mode will at least prevent bradycardia even if the electromyographic potentials reset the stimulation cycle. Another solution, which may also help with extra-cardiac stimulation, is to change from unipolar to bipolar pacing in systems that have this facility.

Atrial pacemakers require a higher sensitivity, because the atrial electrogram is usually of lower amplitude than its ventricular counterpart, and a longer refractory period to avoid sensing the far-field ventricular electrogram. A multiprogrammable generator can be adjusted for use as either an atrial or ventricular pacemaker.

In dual chamber pacing systems, prolongation of the atrial refractory period may prevent endless loop tachycardia. Sometimes endless loop tachycardia can be prevented by reducing sensitivity of the atrial channel so that the atrial electrogram during sinus rhythm is sensed but the atrial electrogram resulting from retrograde conduction, which is usually of lower amplitude, is not detected. In patients with sick sinus syndrome, reprogramming from DDD to DDI or DVI modes will prevent endless loop tachycardia. Alteration from DDD to VVI may be required should atrial fibrillation develop.

Pacemaker clinic

Patients with implanted pacemakers should regularly attend a follow-up clinic. The main purposes are to check that the pacemaker is working satisfactorily; to ensure that there are no pacing complications; to detect impending battery depletion so that generator replacement can be carried out before the patient is at risk; and to maintain a record of patients' locations should a recall of a particular generator or lead be necessary.

The main indicator of impending battery depletion is a reduction in the stimulation rate which has to be measured precisely during fixed rate pacing usually initiated by placing a magnet over the pacemaker. Each type of pacemaker has its own characteristic 'end of life rate': it is usually in the order of a 5–10% reduction of the 'beginning of life' rate.

Intracardiac EGM	A IEGM	
Intracardiac EGM Gain	2.5	mv/div
Chart Speed	25.0	mm/sec

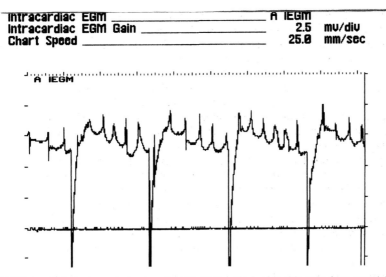

Figure 16.17 Intra-atrial electrogram showing atrial fibrillation obtained by telemetry from an atrial pacing lead in a patient in whom there was doubt as to the atrial rhythm from the surface electrogram

Some pulse generators have the facility to transmit data to the programmer, i.e. telemetry. Information about how the pacemaker has been programmed, battery status, stimulation and sensing thresholds, lead and battery impedance, patient details and even intracardiac electrograms can be obtained (Figure 16.17).

Electromagnetic interference

External electromagnetic interference may be sensed by demand pacemakers and cause either inhibition or reversion to the fixed-rate mode, but the pacemaker will not be damaged. The many sources include electric motors in household devices, internal combustion engines, microwave ovens, radio transmitters, theft and weapon detection systems, arc welding apparatus and radar.

In practice, very few problems are encountered and patients should be reassured that the risks are minimal. Clearly, if a patient feels dizzy near electrical equipment they should quickly walk away from it. If a patient's work brings him into close proximity with strong sources of electromagnetic interference a bipolar pacemaker should be implanted.

Cardioversion may cause pacemaker damage but this should be prevented if the paddles are at least 15 cm from the generator and preferably are positioned so they are at right angles to the pacing system. Pacemaker function should be checked after the procedure.

Diathermy may damage a pacemaker, cause inappropriate inhibition or possibly precipitate ventricular fibrillation. These risks can be avoided if the active electrode is kept at least 15 cm from the generator and the indifferent electrode sited as far away as possible so that its dipole is perpendicular to the pacing system. The pulse should be monitored so that diathermy could be interrupted if prolonged inhibition occurred.

Radiation for diagnostic purposes will not affect a pacemaker but therapeutic levels may cause damage. The pacemaker should be shielded, and if this is not possible re-siting of the generator should be considered.

Limited experience with magnetic resonance imaging indicates that all pacemakers will revert to fixed-rate mode and some will pace at a dangerously fast rate.

Short-wave diathermy can cause pacemaker inhibition.

Advice on practical matters

Patients should be encouraged to lead a normal life. It may be prudent to avoid contact sports because of the risk of damage to the pacemaker or pacemaker site.

In the UK, the presence of complete heart block should be notified to the Licensing Centre and driving should not be permitted. Patients may resume driving 1 month after implantation of a pacemaker provided its function is checked regularly. Heavy goods and public service vehicle drivers may continue to hold a licence provided they are free of symptoms, the pacemaker was implanted to prevent bradycardia and there are no other disqualifying conditions. Annual attendance at a pacemaker clinic is required.

There are no problems with air travel but patients should carry details about their pacemaker in case the pacemaker activates an airport metal detector and in case a pacing problem occurs while abroad.

A pacemaker must be explanted before cremation to avoid explosion.

Main points

- Long-term pacing is indicated in almost all cases of symptomatic bradycardia and should also be considered in asymptomatic patients with second- or third-degree AV block or long pauses in sinus node activity.
- Ventricular demand pacing prevents normal AV synchrony and does not permit a chronotropic response to exercise.
- Loss of normal AV synchrony during ventricular demand pacing may cause symptomatic hypotension (pacemaker syndrome) and can be prevented by atrial or AV sequential pacing.
- Absence of a chronotropic response to exercise can markedly reduce exercise tolerance. Atrial synchronized ventricular pacing and rate response systems sensitive to physiological parameters such as vibration, QT interval and respiration can facilitate a chronotropic response to exercise.
- The modern pacemaker is small, reliable and has a long battery life. Pacemaker infection is the commonest reason for re-operation. Many other complications can be resolved without operation if the pacemaker is programmable.

17

Ambulatory ECG monitoring

Continuous ECG recording
 Clinical applications
  Anti-arrhythmic therapy

'Normal' findings
Artefacts
Infrequent symptoms

Continuous ECG recording

The standard resting electrogram records the heart rhythm for no more than 30 s and is, therefore, not suitable for detecting intermittent disturbances in heart rhythm.

Ambulatory ECG monitoring is an invaluable diagnostic tool. The technique consists of continuously recording the ECG, usually for a period of 24 hours, using a portable battery-operated tape recorder which is worn on a belt at the waist. If appropriate, the patient can be fully ambulant, carrying out his or her normal day-to-day activities.

The electrocardiogram is recorded by means of two electrodes applied to areas of thoroughly cleaned skin. Usually one electrode is placed over the manubrium sterni and the other electrode over the V5 chest lead position. As an alternative a modified V1 lead can be obtained by placing one electrode over the V1 chest lead position and the other electrode beneath the lateral part of the left clavicle.

Some systems allow simultaneous recording of two leads. This increases diagnostic accuracy and aids in the detection of artefact which is unlikely to appear on both leads at the same time. Furthermore, sometimes one lead will not reveal important diagnostic information while another will.

The tape recording is analysed in less than an hour by replaying it at 60–100 times real-time. Playback systems have facilities for printing out selected portions of the recording on ECG paper at standard speed. Most recording systems can automatically detect bradycardias, tachycardias and ectopic beats, though in practice an operator has to supervise the analysis.

Clinical applications

Ambulatory ECG monitoring enables the detection and diagnosis of intermittent disorders of cardiac rhythm and may thus elucidate the cause of symptoms such as syncope, palpitation and chest pain.

The technique is most valuable when the patient actually experiences his usual symptoms during an ECG recording. The patient should be instructed to record the time of onset of his symptoms so that these can be correlated with the heart rhythm at that time. With some recorders the patient can operate an event marker which indicates the onset of symptoms on the tape.

Even when the patient does not experience symptoms during a recording, rhythm abnormalities of diagnostic significance may be detected. Obviously, if the patient does not experience symptoms during the recording and no rhythm abnormalities are found, an arrhythmic cause for the patient's symptoms is not excluded. In the absence of symptoms, the finding of a minor abnormality of rhythm does not rule out a more major rhythm disturbance being responsible for the patient's complaints.

It may sometimes be necessary to record several tapes to obtain diagnostic information.

The technique has demonstrated that in patients with syncope but a normal routine ECG, sinus arrest is often, and complete AV block occasionally, the cause.

Anti-arrhythmic therapy

Ambulatory monitoring is of some value in assessing a patient's response to therapy. For example, not uncommonly a tape recording will reveal frequent ventricular arrhythmias in spite of the use of an anti-arrhythmic agent. One problem in using ambulatory monitoring to assess therapy is that there is a marked spontaneous variation in the frequency of arrhythmias and so on the basis of one tape, absence or improvement in arrhythmia may not necessarily be a consequence of drug therapy.

More importantly, ambulatory electrocardiography may reveal a drug's pro-arrhythmic effect.

'Normal' findings

Sinus bradycardia, short pauses due to sino-atrial block and AV Wenkebach block can occur in normal people during sleep and should not be regarded as evidence of conduction tissue disease. These rhythms may also occur during the day in young people with high vagal tone.

Whereas a routine 12-lead electrocardiogram records approximately 60 heart beats, a normal 24-hour tape recording is likely to contain at least 90 000 beats. Thus ambulatory electrocardiography is a very much more sensitive tool than a standard recording. For example, the finding of a single ventricular ectopic beat on a routine ECG suggests a much higher frequency than a hundred ectopic beats on a 24-hour tape. In fact, studies of apparently normal people using ambulatory electrocardiography have shown that unifocal ventricular extrasystoles occur quite commonly, as do supraventricular ectopic beats. The frequency of ventricular ectopic beats increases with age. Some studies have also found very short runs of relatively slow ventricular tachycardia in apparently normal young subjects.

Artefacts

A number of technical problems during ambulatory electrocardiography can result in what appear to be arrhythmias to the unwary.

If the tape speed slows for any reason, complexes will appear closer together and mimic tachycardia. However, the duration of each ventricular complex will be shorter than normal and this should alert the observer to the likelihood of artefact. Conversely, if the tape runs too fast, apparent bradycardia with broader than normal complexes will result.

Not infrequently, a lead will become disconnected during a recording: since no activity is being recorded the ECG will appear as a straight line and mimic sinus arrest. Furthermore, sometimes an electrical connection can intermittently fail, resulting in repeated episodes of apparent sinus arrest. However, if a lead becomes disconnected it may do so at any point in the cardiac cycle, and it is unlikely that the onset of 'asystole' will arise after the ventricular T wave as it would if sinus arrest were real. If the onset of sinus arrest does occur during the inscription of an atrial or ventricular complex, artefact can be assumed.

Occasionally, artefact can produce an apparent tachycardia but close inspection will reveal that normal QRS complexes are 'walking through' the tachycardia.

Infrequent symptoms

Patients with infrequent symptoms such as palpitation are unlikely to experience an episode during a 24-hour recording. A very useful and relatively inexpensive device (cardio-memo recorder) enables a patient to record the electrocardiogram for 30 s during symptoms. The patient can carry the device around until an attack occurs. He or she then applies the device to the chest wall and initiates the recording which is stored in a memory and can be replayed directly or transmitted via the telephone into an ECG machine. Recently, a similar device which is worn like a wrist-watch has become available.

Clearly, the device is not suitable for the investigation of episodes that disable the patient to the extent that they cannot activate the recorder. It is very important to explain to the patient precisely when and how to use the recorder.

Main points

- Ambulatory electrocardiography is very useful for the investigation of syncope, near-syncope, palpitation and other symptoms thought to be due to an arrhythmia when routine electrocardiography has not provided diagnostic information.
- Artefact can produce apparent arrhythmias but can usually be recognized by careful inspection of the recording.
- Studies in apparently normal subjects have demonstrated that certain rhythm disturbances detected by ambulatory electrocardiography are not of pathological significance.
- For patients with infrequent, non-disabling palpitation, provision of a cardio-memo recorder is the best method of investigation.
- Useful information will be provided from an ambulatory recording if an arrhythmia is demonstrated or if a patient experiences his usual symptoms without a disturbance in rhythm. Clearly if there is no arrhythmia and no symptoms, an episodic arrhythmia has not been excluded.

18

Arrhythmias for interpretation

Examples of a variety of arrhythmias are given. Their interpretations can be found at the end of the chapter. As is often the case in practice, there may be more than one observation to make about each example.

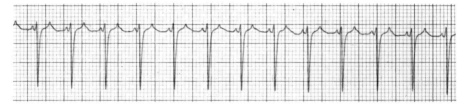

Figure 18.1

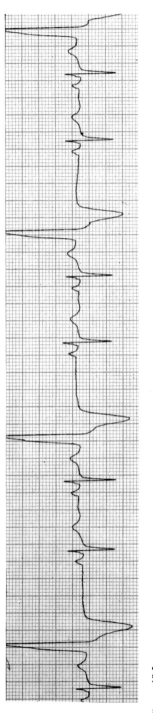

Figure 18.2

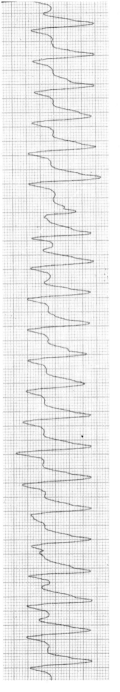

Figure 18.3

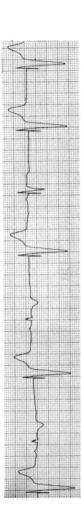

Figure 18.4

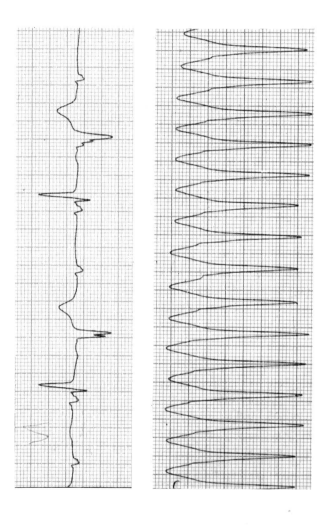

Figure 18.5

Figure 18.6

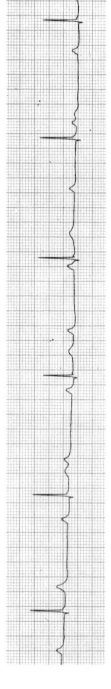

Figure 18.7

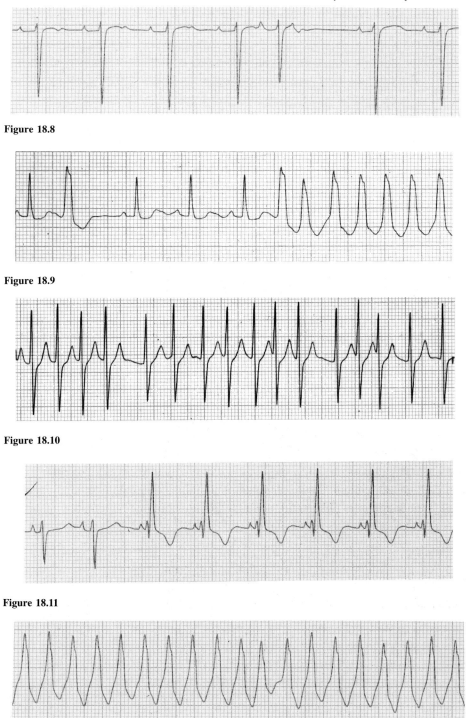

Figure 18.8

Figure 18.9

Figure 18.10

Figure 18.11

Figure 18.12

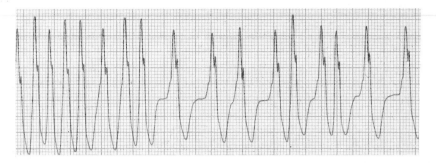

Figure 18.13

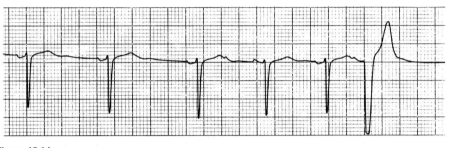

 Figure 18.14

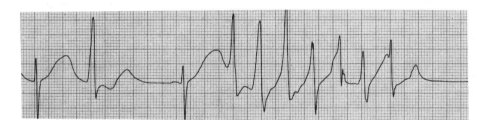

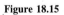**Figure 18.15**

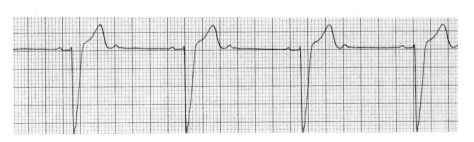

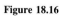**Figure 18.16**

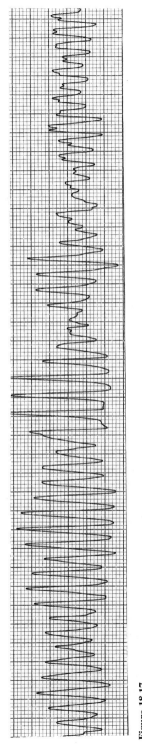

Figure 18.17

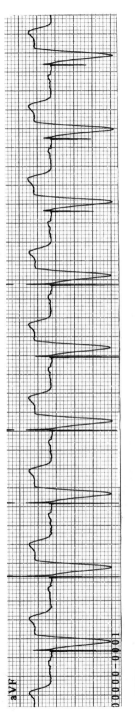

aVF

00000-0001

Figure 18.18

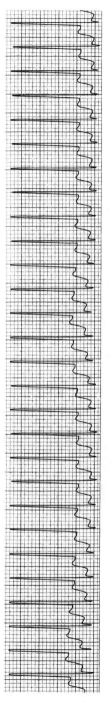

Figure 18.19

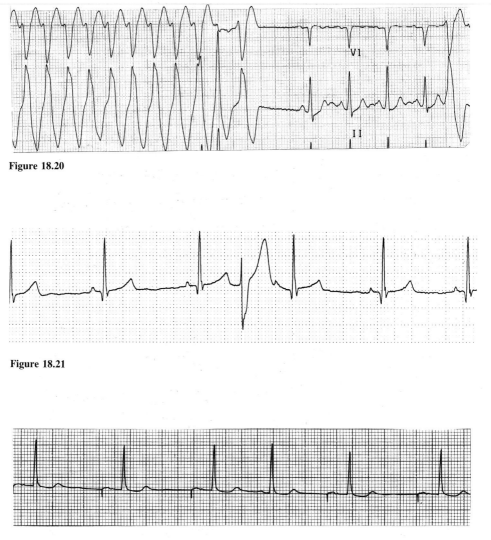

Figure 18.20

Figure 18.21

Figure 18.22

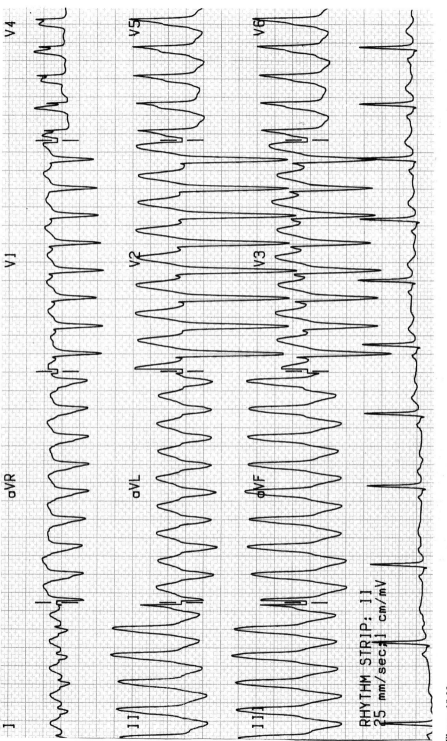

Figure 18.23

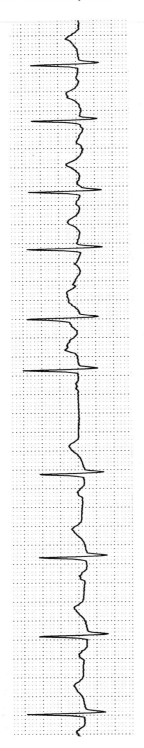

Figure 18.24

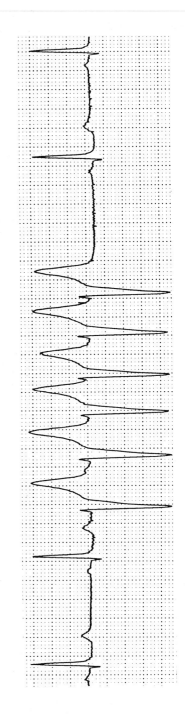

Figure 18.25

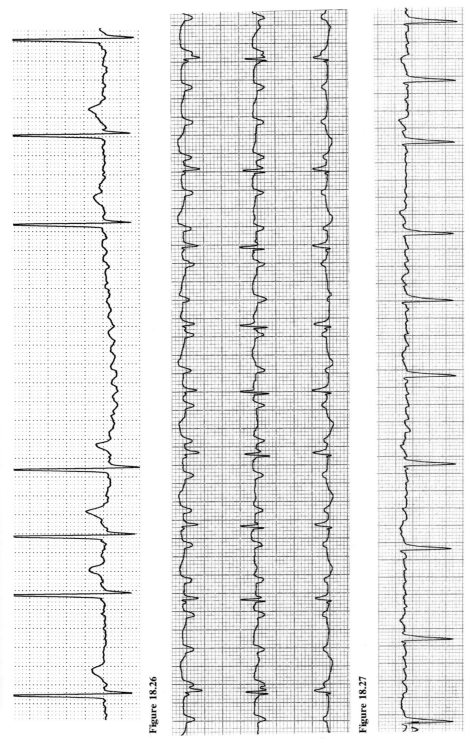

Figure 18.26

Figure 18.27

Figure 18.28

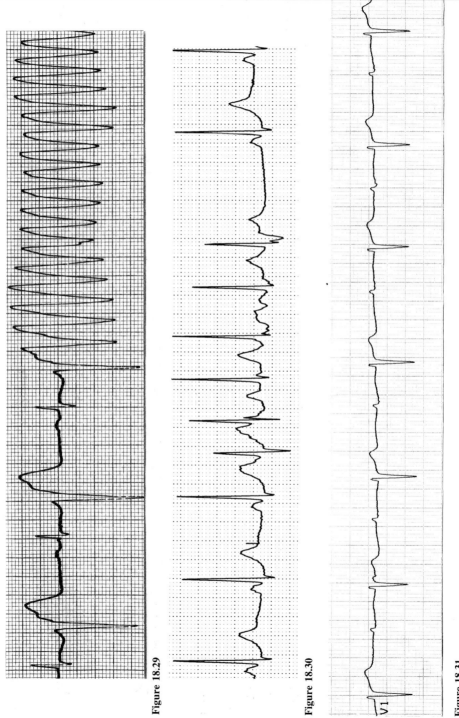

Figure 18.29

Figure 18.30

V1

Figure 18.31

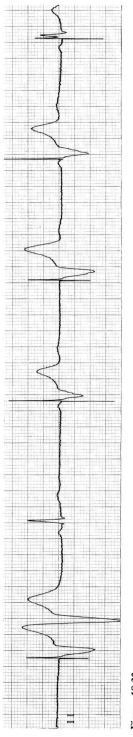

Figure 18.32

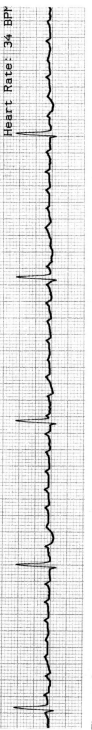
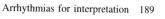

Figure 18.33

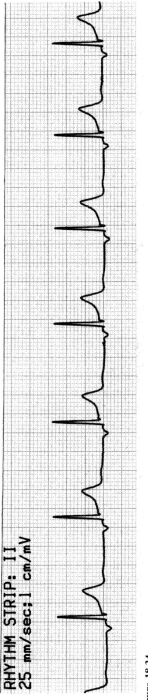

RHYTHM STRIP: II
25 mm/sec; 1 cm/mV

Figure 18.34

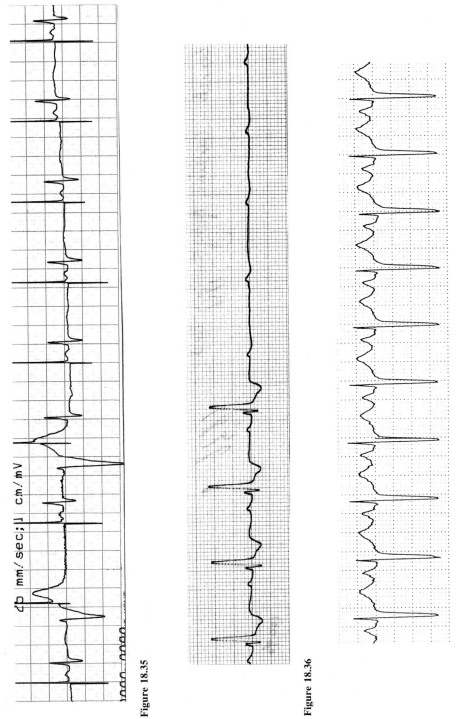

Figure 18.35

Figure 18.36

Figure 18.37

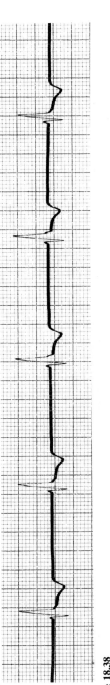

Figure 18.38

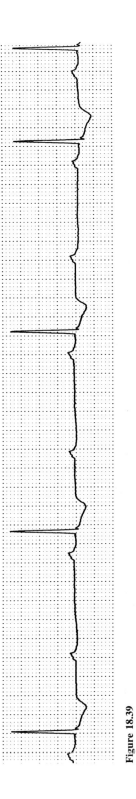

Figure 18.39

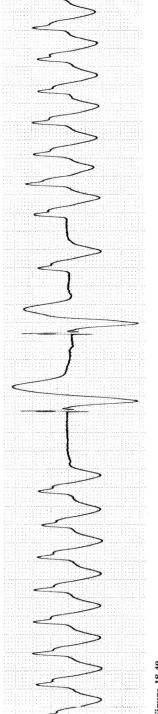

Figure 18.40

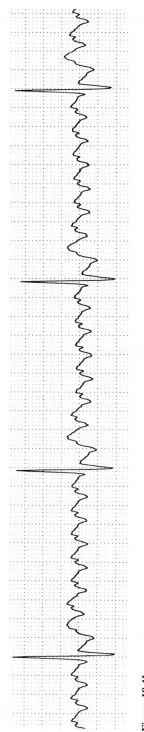

Figure 18.41

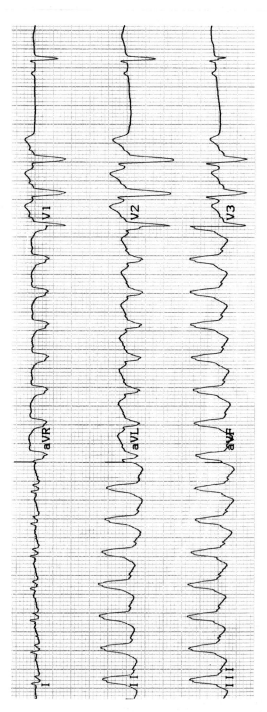

Figure 18.42

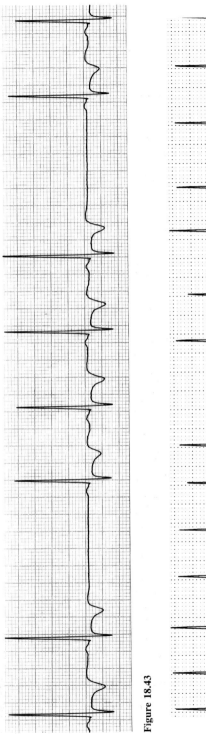

Figure 18.43

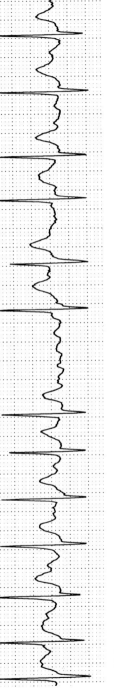

Figure 18.44

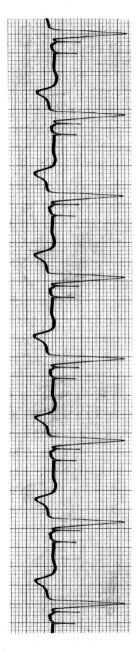

Figure 18.45

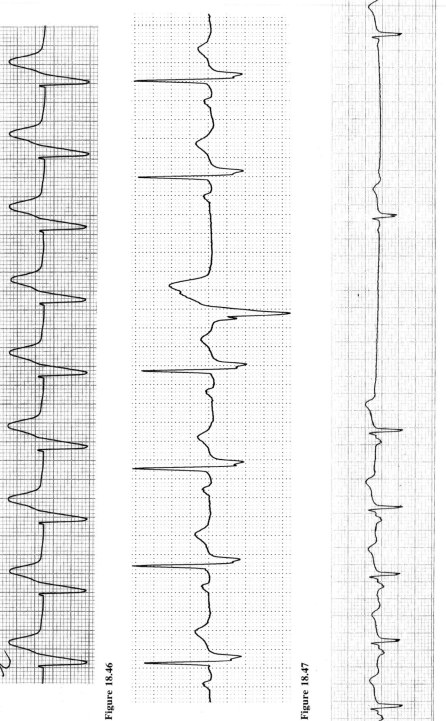

Figure 18.46

Figure 18.47

Figure 18.48

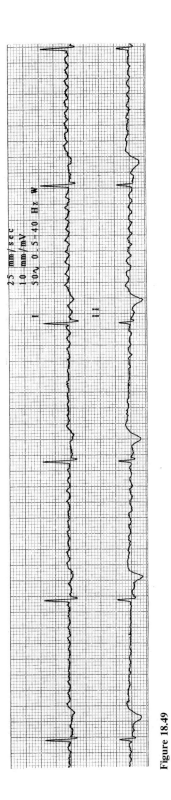

25 mm/sec
10 mm/mV
50 ~ 0.5-40 Hz W

Figure 18.49

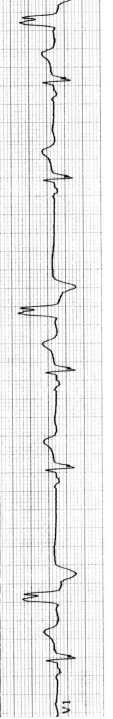
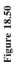

Figure 18.50

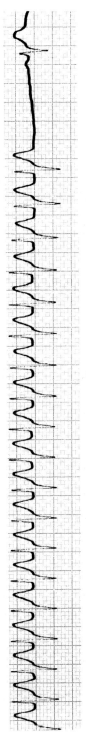

Figure 18.51

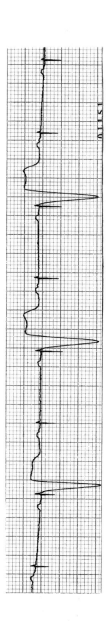

Figure 18.52

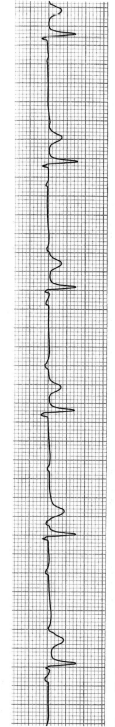

Figure 18.53

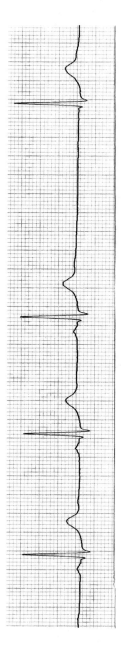

Figure 18.54

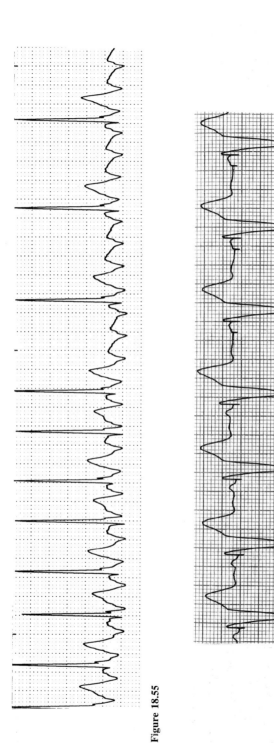

Figure 18.55

Figure 18.56

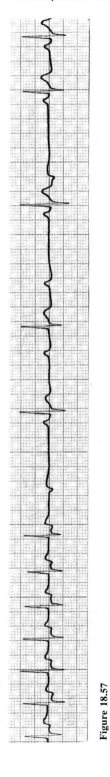

Figure 18.57

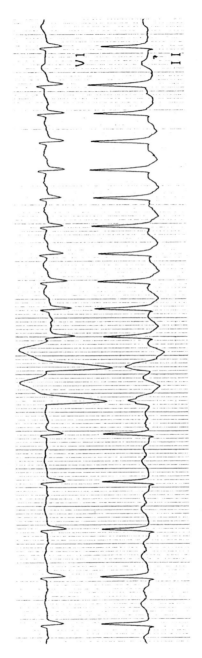

Figure 18.58

Answers

Figure 18.1 Atrial flutter with 2:1 AV block

Figure 18.2 Sinus rhythm with ventricular trigeminy

Figure 18.3 Ventricular tachycardia. The sixteenth complex is a fusion beat

Figure 18.4 Ventricular demand pacemaker inhibited by sinus beats. The sixth complex is a fusion beat

Figure 18.5 2:1 AV block with ventricular ectopic beats

Figure 18.6 Ventricular tachycardia

Figure 18.7 Complete AV block with narrow ventricular complexes

Figure 18.8 Atrial ectopic beat superimposed on T wave of fourth ventricular complex. There is a further atrial ectopic beat superimposed on the T wave of the fifth complex which is not conducted to the ventricles

Figure 18.9 The second ventricular ectopic beat initiates ventricular tachycardia

Figure 18.10 Atrial fibrillation with rapid ventricular response

Figure 18.11 After two normally conducted sinus beats there is right bundle branch block (lead V1)

Figure 18.12 Ventricular tachycardia with a fusion beat.

Figure 18.13 Atrial fibrillation. Configuration of ventricular complexes suggests Wolff–Parkinson–White syndrome

Figure 18.14 Atrial ectopic beats superimposed on third and fifth ventricular T waves. First ectopic beat is not conducted; the second is conducted to the ventricles with left bundle branch block

Figure 18.15 Sinus bradycardia with long QT interval and short episode of torsade de pointes tachycardia

Figure 18.16 2:1 AV block

Figure 18.17 Ventricular fibrillation

Figure 18.18 Atrial synchronized ventricular pacing

Figure 18.19 AV re-entrant tachycardia

Figure 18.20 Termination of ventricular tachycardia followed by four sinus beats and a ventricular ectopic beat

Figure 18.21 The fourth ventricular complex is an interpolated ventricular ectopic beat

Figure 18.22 Atrial pacing. After three paced beats, a sinus beat inhibits the pacemaker

Figure 18.23 12-lead ECG showing right ventricular outflow tract tachycardia. Sinus rhythm has returned at time of recording rhythm strip

Figure 18.24 Atrial fibrillation after five sinus beats

Figure 18.25 Short episode of ventricular tachycardia

Figure 18.26 Atrial fibrillation with long pause in ventricular activity

Figure 18.27 Atrial tachycardia with AV block

Figure 18.28 Atrial fibrillation

Figure 18.29 Ventricular tachycardia initiated by third ventricular ectopic beat

Figure 18.30 Paroxysmal atrial fibrillation

Figure 18.31 First-degree AV block. PR interval = 0.46 s

Figure 18.32 Ventricular demand pacing at 40 beats/minute. Ventricular ectopic after first paced beat. Last complex is a fusion beat

Figure 18.33 Atrial flutter with complete AV block

Figure 18.34 Junctional rhythm

Figure 18.35 Atrial pacing. There are two ventricular ectopic beats which are of course not sensed by pacemaker

Figure 18.36 Ventricular asystole after four sinus beats conducted with right bundle branch block

Figure 18.37 Sinus tachycardia

Figure 18.38 Junctional rhythm

Figure 18.39 Mobitz II AV block

Figure 18.40 Two paced ventricular beats preceded and succeeded by ventricular tachycardia

Figure 18.41 Atrial flutter with high-degree AV block

Figure 18.42 Ventricular tachycardia with retrograde atrial activation. Sinus rhythm returns at end of ECG.

Figure 18.43 Two episodes of second-degree sinoatrial block

Figure 18.44 Atrial fibrillation

Figure 18.45 AV sequential pacing

Figure 18.46 Idioventricular rhythm

Figure 18.47 Single ventricular ectopic beat. First-degree AV block

Figure 18.48 Junctional rhythm followed by sinus arrest and then sinus bradycardia

Figure 18.49 Atrial fibrillation and complete AV block

Figure 18.50 Ventricular trigeminy

Figure 18.51 Termination of AV re-entrant tachycardia

Figure 18.52 Ventricular pacing with intermittent failure to capture

Figure 18.53 Complete AV block

Figure 18.54 Sinus arrest followed by junctional escape beat

Figure 18.55 Atrial flutter with varying AV conduction

Figure 18.56 Atrial synchronized and then AV sequential pacing, i.e. DDD pacemaker

Figure 18.57 Complete heart block following termination of supraventricular tachycardia – suggesting that adenosine has been given

Figure 18.58 Onset of AV re-entrant tachycardia following couplet of ventricular ectopic beats

Index